SpringerBriefs in Applied Sciences and Technology

Series editor

Janusz Kacprzyk, Polish Academy of Sciences, Systems Research Institute, Warsaw, Poland

SpringerBriefs present concise summaries of cutting-edge research and practical applications across a wide spectrum of fields. Featuring compact volumes of 50–125 pages, the series covers a range of content from professional to academic. Typical publications can be:

- A timely report of state-of-the art methods
- An introduction to or a manual for the application of mathematical or computer techniques
- A bridge between new research results, as published in journal articles
- A snapshot of a hot or emerging topic
- An in-depth case study
- A presentation of core concepts that students must understand in order to make independent contributions

SpringerBriefs are characterized by fast, global electronic dissemination, standard publishing contracts, standardized manuscript preparation and formatting guidelines, and expedited production schedules.

On the one hand, **SpringerBriefs in Applied Sciences and Technology** are devoted to the publication of fundamentals and applications within the different classical engineering disciplines as well as in interdisciplinary fields that recently emerged between these areas. On the other hand, as the boundary separating fundamental research and applied technology is more and more dissolving, this series is particularly open to trans-disciplinary topics between fundamental science and engineering.

Indexed by EI-Compendex and Springerlink.

More information about this series at http://www.springer.com/series/8884

Roman Trobec · Ivan Tomašić
Aleksandra Rashkovska · Matjaž Depolli
Viktor Avbelj

Body Sensors
and Electrocardiography

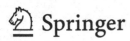

Roman Trobec
Department of Communication Systems
Jožef Stefan Institute
Ljubljana
Slovenia

Matjaž Depolli
Department of Communication Systems
Jožef Stefan Institute
Ljubljana
Slovenia

Ivan Tomašić
Division of Intelligent Future Technologies
Mälardalen University
Västerås
Sweden

Viktor Avbelj
Department of Communication Systems
Jožef Stefan Institute
Ljubljana
Slovenia

Aleksandra Rashkovska
Department of Communication Systems
Jožef Stefan Institute
Ljubljana
Slovenia

ISSN 2191-530X   ISSN 2191-5318   (electronic)
SpringerBriefs in Applied Sciences and Technology
ISBN 978-3-319-59338-8   ISBN 978-3-319-59340-1   (eBook)
DOI 10.1007/978-3-319-59340-1

Library of Congress Control Number: 2017944172

Printed on acid-free paper

This Springer imprint is published by Springer Nature
The registered company is Springer International Publishing AG
The registered company address is: Gewerbestrasse 11, 6330 Cham, Switzerland

To all who make our lives worthwhile.

Preface

This monograph presents a comprehensive overview of electrocardiography from the aspect of wireless and mobile monitoring and its potential for personalized health management. Personalized healthcare diagnostic procedures and treatments are tailored to individual patients and therefore more efficient. The main advantage of wireless and mobile ECG systems, compared to traditional ECG devices, is the ability to generate ECG measurements by a single or a few wireless and non-obstructive personal sensors. In addition, the sensors are potentially multi-functional in the sense that, besides ECG, they can also measure other physiological and biochemical parameters, e.g., heart rate, respiration, ballistocardiogram, blood pressure, blood oxygen saturation, body temperature, posture, or physical activities, thus providing insight into the medical status of the monitored person.

Body sensors can be used for both inpatient and outpatient monitoring, thus enabling cardiac monitoring and diagnostic decisions to be made during normal everyday activities. Since the employment of remote and outpatient monitoring technologies also reduces the costs of health care, it is evident that such an approach could become widely applicable in the near future—for patients and those who care for their health. The spectrum of book topics covers the implementation and efficient application of user-friendly mHealth systems. The target audience comprises biomedical engineers, medical doctors, students, industrial experts, and health managers developing mHealth solutions. The book may be interesting and useful also for the wider public in the parts where basic principles of mobile monitoring and their benefits for users are presented.

We are grateful to all our colleagues who have contributed to this book through discussions, clinical work, or by reading the material, in particular to Prof. Borut Geršak, M.D., Ph.D., to Assist. Prof. Jurij Matija Kališnik, M.D., Ph.D., and many other medical professionals who have collaborated in our joint projects. Many thanks to Dr. Monika Kapus-Kolar for carefully proofreading the text and resolving many formal and linguistic inconsistencies. We are indebted to the Jožef Stefan Institute for support and constructive research spirit. We acknowledge the financial support from the Slovenian Research Agency under the grant P2-0095 and the EkoSMART project, grant No. C3330-16-529007, financed by the European

Regional Development Fund. Additionally, Ivan Tomašić thanks the Swedish Knowledge Foundation (KKS) for their support through projects CCOPD, reference number: 20160029, and the Embedded Sensor Systems for Health research profile.

Ljubljana, Slovenia   Roman Trobec
March 2017   Ivan Tomašić
                                                            Aleksandra Rashkovska
                                                                  Matjaž Depolli
                                                                    Viktor Avbelj

Contents

Acronyms

AECG	Abdominal ECG
AF	Atrial fibrillation
AP	Action potential
AV	Atrioventricular
BLE	Bluetooth low energy
BPM	Beats per minute
BSM	Body surface mapping
CC	Correlation coefficient
CHCL	Community Health Centre Ljubljana
COPD	Chronic obstructive pulmonary disease
DL	Differential lead
ECG	Electrocardiogram
EDR	ECG-derived respiration
EEG	Electroencephalogram
EMA	Exponential moving average
EMG	Electromyogram
FECG	Fetal ECG
FLOPS	Floating point operations per second
HR	Heart rate
HRV	Heart rate variability
I	Inferior
ICT	Information and communication technologies
ILR	Implantable loop recorder
L	Left
LA	Left arm
LL	Left leg
MECG	Multichannel electrocardiography
MEMS	Micro-electromechanical systems
MEWS	Modified early warning score
mHealth	Mobile health

MWBS	Multifunctional wireless body sensors
NN	Neural network
PAB	Premature atrial beat
PCARD	Personal device for CARDiac activity
PDA	Personal digital assistant
POAF	Postoperative atrial fibrillation
R	Right
RA	Right arm
RMSD	Root-mean-square distance
RSA	Respiratory sinus arrhythmia
S	Superior
sEMG	Surface electromyography
SIM	Simulation center
SN	Sinus node
SR	Sinus rhythm
UMCL	University Medical Centre Ljubljana
VCG	Vectorcardiography
VES	Ventricular extra systole
WBS	Wireless body sensor
WCT	Wilson central terminal
WHO	World Health Organization

Chapter 1
Introduction

Abstract The motivation and goals for the development of mobile health solutions are presented. Short history and background of the electrocardiography provide basic principles and facts related to the heart activity and elucidate the path from the measurement of conventional electrocardiogram to the monitoring of the heart by wireless body sensors. A bipolar differential lead is introduced, which has enabled the implementation of a small body sensor for capturing electric potential differences on the skin. The chapter concludes with guidelines on how to read this book and with a short overview of all book chapters.

1.1 Historical Evolution of Electrocardiography

Electrocardiogram (ECG) is a recording of electrical activity of the heart by using electrodes usually placed on the skin. High-quality ECG was first measured by Willem Einthoven at the beginning of the 20th century with his invention of the string galvanometer. The whole ECG machine weighted about 300 kg (Fig. 1.1a). Today, a range of ECG devices are used in medicine, from the well-known standard 12-lead ECG (Fig. 1.1b), where wires are connected to electrodes placed on 10 locations on the body, to multichannel ECG body surface mapping systems [1] (Fig. 1.1c), to the Holter monitor (first introduced by Norman J. Holter, 1961) [2], where a reduced number of electrodes are connected with wires to a small portable recorder that obtains continuous ECG measurement throughout several days (Fig. 1.1d), and finally to the (wireless) implantable loop recorder that measures ECG for more than a year and weighs only 17 g [3]. The last case is an invasive ECG measurement where a special device is inserted under the skin.

The use of the standard 12-lead ECG and the use of multichannel ECG systems are mostly limited to short-term monitoring in a resting position. On the other hand, the Holter monitor represents the most frequently utilized option for ECG monitoring that lasts for several days. Its main limitations are the relatively short duration of the recordings (14 days) and the discomfort from the cabling and the device during long-term use. The advantages of the implantable loop recorder include the capacity for long-term ECG monitoring and no discomfort for the patient, as there are no external

© The Author(s) 2018
R. Trobec et al., *Body Sensors and Electrocardiography*, SpringerBriefs
in Applied Sciences and Technology, DOI 10.1007/978-3-319-59340-1_1

(a)   (b)

(c)   (d)

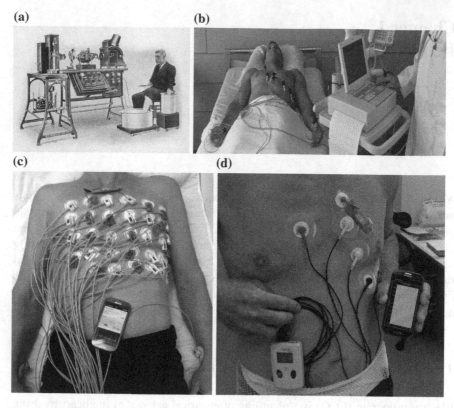

Fig. 1.1 ECG devices over time. **a** The first ECG device. **b** 12-lead ECG from Schiller. Picture taken from the company's web site http://www.schiller.ch (accessed on Jan 25, 2017). **c** Multichannel ECG. **d** Holter monitor compared to an ECG body sensor

parts. The negative aspects include the necessity for an invasive procedure at the time of implantation and extraction of the device. The capacity for ECG recording is limited to several recordings with a duration of a couple of minutes. Afterwards, if the patient does not visit the medical office, older recordings are overwritten.

Long-term ECG monitoring with a Holter monitor has been used in medicine since the 60s of the last century. The development of electronics has enabled these devices to be made small and to record high-quality ECG signals from one or more leads. The measurements are made available for detailed analysis after one or more days of recording. Since the recordings made with a Holter monitor are intended for diagnosis in medicine [2], the quality of the recordings is extremely important, which is mostly determined by the quality of the contact between the electrodes and the skin. On the other hand, the development of telecommunications in recent years enabled wireless data transmission [4] from miniature sensor devices to nearby personal terminals (smartphone, tablet) that have access to the Internet. This in turn enabled provision of a wide range of mobile health services, from patient monitoring in hospitals [5], through remote medical support, and finally to sports and entertainment. Research efforts are focused on the development of devices and instruments which are smaller, simple to use and reliable. The trends in recent years are towards wireless body sensors applied for patient monitoring [6, 7].

1.2 Motivation and Goals

The aim for constant improvements in medical treatments and more effective health care from the side of medical professionals, the intention for higher quality of life, mobility and awareness about own health from the side of patients and wider population, and finally, a quest for sustainable budget costs spent for the public health care are the three most important drivers for increased engagement of information and communication technologies (ICT) in the health care system. It can be expected that new generations of users, potential patients and medical practitioners will accept new technologies on a day-to-day basis.

The mobile health (mHealth), which enables telemonitoring, telecare, teleconsultations and other distant services, can be regarded as a new way of supporting clinical health care in the era of infrastructure supporting the mobile community. Mobile communications are accessible almost everywhere, either by smart electronic devices, which have become personal necessities of life, or by other public communication options like the Internet. The wearable wireless sensors have advanced far enough to provide reliable physiological readings for health management.

The technological challenges for mHealth are well known. The communication infrastructure should interact with users in an unobtrusive way—through a small number of small wireless devices that are able to record multiple vital signs during the every-day user's activity. The recorded data should be reliably and safely transferred to a personal device, either a smartphone or a tablet, where they are temporarily stored, visualized and analyzed. Finally, the measurements should be transferred to a computer (preferably a Cloud-based computer server) to provide authorized access to medical professionals who can use computer supported analysis and diagnostics. The key weakness of already implemented approaches is that they mainly focus on the technology, while the importance of the acceptance of ICT devices by users and health care practitioners is largely neglected. Therefore, despite the world of ubiquitous mHealth enabling ICT devices, there is a lack of widely accepted mHealth solutions.

Many branches of medicine, today implemented on a face-to-face basis, can be taken over by mHealth capabilities, i.e., consulting, monitoring, diagnostics, etc. The measured data, through periods of several days or weeks or longer, can be visualized and preliminary analyzed with a dedicated program on a personal computer. The program should generate condensed reports for the medical practitioners, supporting further decisions related to users' health management. The whole system should stimulate a proactive engagement and care of users for their own health and wellbeing. A conceptual scheme of an mHealth platform based on multifunctional body sensors,

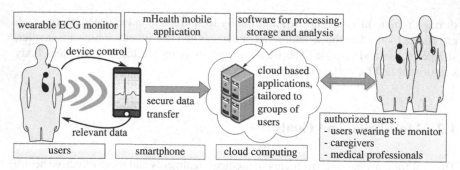

Fig. 1.2 Conceptual scheme of an mHealth platform based on ICT technologies

mobile technologies and communications, and safe storage and processing servers, is shown in Fig. 1.2. Either healthy users or patients (leftmost) are equipped with ECG sensors that serve as heart monitoring devices. The ECG sensor communicates wirelessly with a smartphone to establish the communication protocol and, most of the time, to transmit the measured ECG data stream. The users interact with the smartphone and not directly with the body sensor. Both types of interaction, the control of the sensor and the transfer of relevant data to the smartphone, are important in an mHealth system. The smartphone in turn transmits the measured data to a computer Cloud that can store the huge amount of data. Finally, the data on the Cloud can be accessed, analyzed and visualized by authorized users, including medical practitioners, caregivers and the patients themselves.

Multifunctional body sensors are the key elements of the mHealth platform. Even though many are already available, they must be perpetually upgraded and improved to be widely accepted by the users. The first reason is that they are in an intimate contact with the users and, therefore, their formative design and unobtrusiveness are crucial. The second reason is that they record vital users' signals, which have to enable an accurate evidence-based medicine. The rest of the ICT technology devices in the mHealth platform are already quite mature and available on the market.

An ultimate goal of the ICT designers is to develop a multifunctional body sensorthat would primarily measure the surface potential difference between proximal electrodes near the heart, which is the ECG. Besides ECG, other features can be extracted from the measured potential differences, such as brain activity with electroencephalogram (EEG), muscular activity with electromyogram (EMG) or ECG-derived respiration (EDR). The sensor should also detect information about the environmental conditions in which the measurements were recorded, such as movements, light, humidity or temperature, thus providing information that allows for ambient intelligence. Even though we promote multifunctionality, in the sense that a single body sensor is able to measure different signals, we will focus in this book on the ECG measurements.

1.3 ECG Basics

A coordinated action of all myocardial cells is possible because of their ability to "communicate". Each excitable cardiac cell can be activated by an influx of positive ions into the cell, which causes reduction of the transmembrane potential up to a threshold where sudden inrush of sodium ions (Na+) through the cell membrane results in a fast depolarization of the cell. As the cells are interconnected by discs with ion permeable channels, the depolarization wave goes from cell to cell. The depolarization of the cells, which have myofibrils (molecular "stepper motors"), causes a flow of other ions (Ca2+, K+, Cl+) and the main result is a reduction of the length of these cells by usage of chemical energy. The reduction of the length is a mechanical force that results in pumping action of the heart. The depolarized cell returns into its previous polarized state by moving the ions through the cell membrane by active processes where chemical energy is used again. These processes cause repolarization after which the cell is prepared for the next heartbeat. The depolarization and repolarization of the cell is called action potential (AP) [8].

As explained above, the chemical energy is used for the mechanical work and for the communication among the cardiac cells. As the left ventricle pushes the blood to the highest pressure, the prevailing part of the energy goes to this chamber, because it has the largest mass among the heart chambers. For efficient mechanical work of a heart chamber, all its cells have to start the contraction near the same time. Even more, the atria must contract before ventricles. This complex task is resolved by the differentiation of cardiac cells for three different tasks: pacemaking and delaying (sinoatrial and atrioventricular node), fast spread of the depolarization wave from the nodes to the chambers (His-Purkinje system), and contraction for the mechanical work. All these functions should be accomplished in a wide range of heart rates and blood flow rates, which goes from about five liters per minute up to 6 times higher. These tasks are fulfilled with: (a) adaptive mechanisms inside cardiac cells, (b) the local autonomic nervous system of the heart, (c) the autonomic nervous system outside of the heart, directly to cardiac nodes and to other cardiac cells, and (d) by hormones circulating in the blood. When these tasks are not done effectively, the heart loses efficiency and also becomes vulnerable to arrhythmia, which generally means loss of precisely coordinated actions.

All ion currents in the heart produce potential differences on the cardiac surface. These differences are momentarily transferred to the whole body by the ion currents in the tissues outside the heart and also on the body surface where ECG is normally measured. The potential differences are measured between two electrodes that are fixed on the skin. The electrical contact between the electrode and the skin is provided by a conductive liquid or gel that is coated on the bottom side of the electrode. The number of body electrodes could be as small as two, as in modern mHealth devices, and as large as several hundreds, as in a multichannel ECG. The conventional 12-lead ECG has been known since 1942, when augmented limb leads aVR, aVL and aVF were introduced, but is still used as a golden standard for clinical cardiac diagnoses.

The knowledge for the 12-lead ECG interpretation has accumulated over the years, which has an important impact on the everyday cardiology practice.

The standard 12-lead ECG consists of three bipolar leads: I, II and III, which measure the surface body potential differences in the vertical plane, i.e., the voltage between pairs of electrodes placed on the limbs. For example, lead I measures the voltage between the left arm (LA) and the right arm (RA), hence it reflects the sum of all potential differences in the direction designated with $0°$ angle in the vertical plane, assuming that the heart is the center of the coordinate system. Note that the positive pole of lead I is LA. In the same way, lead II measures the voltage between the left leg (LL) and RA, covering the direction designated with $60°$ angle and with the positive pole on LL. Lead III measures the voltage between LL and LA, thus covers the direction of $120°$, again with the positive pole on LL. Another three leads, aVF, aVL and aVR, are termed as augmented leads. No separate electrodes are needed for the calculation of the augmented leads. They are obtained with a combination of voltages measured on bipolar leads in order to cover the reaming vertical plane directions: $90°$, $-30°$ and $-150°$. The positive poles of the augmented leads are again in directions denoted by standard notation, e.g., aVF covers the sum of potential differences in the direction $90°$, which is the LL. In the same way, the positive poles of aVL and aVR are LA and RA, respectively.

Six precordial leads, V1 to V6, are obtained from electrodes placed on the chest which are referenced to a common potential, termed as Wilson central terminal (WCT). The precordial leads cover six directions in the horizontal plane, from $0°$ to $100°$, in steps of $20°$, starting with V1 on $100°$ and ending with V6 on $0°$. In this way, the precordial leads cover the most important parts of the right and left atria and ventricles. The positive poles of the precordial leads are on the body, in positions of the chest electrodes.

The standardized placement and naming of the 10 electrodes of the conventional 12-lead ECG are shown in the left part of Fig. 1.3. The right part of the same figure shows a closer look on the heart with the corresponding 12 leads (view angles). If the potential differences are captured on all electrodes with an appropriate frequency, e.g. several hundred times per second, we are able to monitor the average magnitudes and directions of the electrical activity of the heart, which are covered by the described 12 leads. The graphs of voltage versus time for each lead, printed on a paper with a millimeter grid background, are presented as a standard 12-lead ECG. A more formal description of the leads can be found in Chap. 5.

A typical ECG signal from lead V5 of the standard 12-lead ECG is shown in Fig. 1.4. The ECG graph includes characteristic shapes and intervals of ECG waves that provide an important diagnostic value obtained from a matured knowledge and tested in clinical praxis. Normal or sinus rhythm produces four typical entities: P wave, QRS complex, T wave and U wave. A sinus heartbeat is initiated in a small area of specialized cells in the right atrium, termed as a sinus node (SN), which starts the atrial depolarization and consequently the contraction of atrial muscles. The P wave corresponds to the depolarization of atrial cells. The atrio-ventricular (AV) node

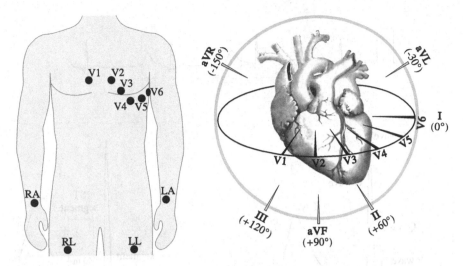

Fig. 1.3 Placement and naming of the 10 electrodes of the conventional 12-lead ECG (*left*), and a closer look on the heart in vertical and horizontal planes through 12 view angles—leads (*right*)

will initiate, after a small delay, the depolarization of the His-Purkinje system, which in the next phase depolarizes the ventricles. The ventricular depolarization is reflected in the QRS complex, composed of three waves: Q, R and S. The QRS complex is much larger in the amplitude than the P wave because the muscular volume of the ventricles is much larger than the volume of the atrial muscle. The repolarization of the ventricles is reflected in the T wave, which is a residual of unbalanced ends of APs in the ventricular cells. Note that a small signal from the repolarization of atria is hidden in the QRS complex. The origin of the U wave is still not known and is most probably related to a mechanical reflection on the change of APs during relaxation of the myocardial cells [9]. U waves are not always visible, but prominent or inverted U waves have clinical importance [10, 11].

The interpretations of ECG reports are performed mainly on the basis of rules. In order to understand the ECG patterns, a few basic assumptions should be respected:

- If the depolarization front of the heart travels more towards the positive electrode, a positive wave is recorded in the ECG.
- If the travel of the depolarization front is more away from the positive electrode, a negative ECG wave is recorded.
- The repolarization of the heart towards the positive electrode results in a negative ECG wave.
- The repolarization of the heart away from the positive electrode results in a positive ECG wave.

The propagation directions of the depolarization and the repolarization are important for the ECG analysis, including damages of the myocardial cells or characterization of arrhythmic events. For example, if the atrial depolarization starts from the right

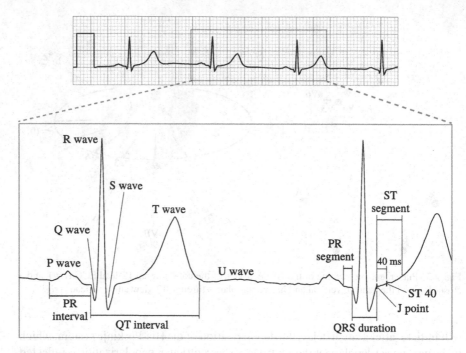

Fig. 1.4 Sinus ECG signal with characteristic ECG waves and their intervals

atrium and propagates to the left, a positive P wave will be observed in lead I, because the depolarization front propagates towards the positive electrode of I, which is on the left arm.

1.4 Differential Lead

The idea for wireless ECG is based on our experiences with 35-channel ECG measurements where the potentials of all leads are referenced to the WCT. The potential difference, by definition the voltage U, between two channels results now in a bipolar ECG signal, which is termed in the following as differential lead, body sensor ECG or simply sensor ECG. The sensor ECG can be measured on the skin with two proximal electrodes. Such a measurement is equivalent to an algebraic difference of voltages from two multichannel leads if the electrodes of the body sensor would be positioned on the same places as the two multichannel electrodes. Because the precordial leads (V1 to V6) of the standard 12-lead ECG are also referenced to the WCT, the V1 and V2 leads can be denoted with voltages U_{V1} and U_{V2}, respectively. If the body sensor electrodes are placed now on the positions of the electrodes V1 and V2, the differential lead, measured with the body sensor, is equivalent to the algebraic difference $U_{V2-V1} = U_{V2} - U_{V1}$. A schematic placement of the sensor electrodes,

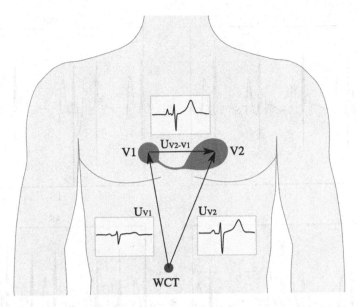

Fig. 1.5 V1 and V2 leads with WCT as a common reference point, and a differential lead from the positions of V1 and V2 electrodes, with the corresponding voltages U_{V1} and U_{V2} (two graphs) and the resulting sensor ECG denoted by U_{V2-V1}

with the negative sensor electrode in the position of the electrode V1 and the positive sensor electrode in the position of the electrode V2, is shown in Fig. 1.5, together with the corresponding schematic ECG signals. The V1 and the V2 ECGs are shown in the left and the right graph, respectively, while the resulting differential lead is shown above the sensor in a separate graph. A more detailed theoretical description of the differential lead is introduced in Chap. 5.

Because the electrodes of a differential lead can be close, e.g., at a distance of 10 cm, we are able to look on them as on a single unit—sensor. It can be equipped with a signal processing electronics, a small low-power radio and a battery, resulting in a small wireless body sensor. One would speculate that such a sensor could become arbitrarily small. However, if the proximal electrodes are too close, the ECG signal also becomes small and the signal-to-noise ratio reaches a level which prevents a reliable use. Based on numerous experiments, we found out that the optimal distance between the differential electrodes is about 8 cm. Because of the requirement for sustainable power consumption, we select 125 samples/s for the signal sampling rate as an optimal compromise for acceptable autonomy of the sensor, which results in once-per-week charging of the built-in battery. The moderate resolution ECG, e.g. 125 Hz, is suitable for long-term personal cardiac activity monitoring, as well as for clinical use. The sensor can be lightweight in design, e.g., with a weight of 20 g, which allows for unobstructed use also during sports activities or during exhaustive physical work. The device can support solutions to every-day problems

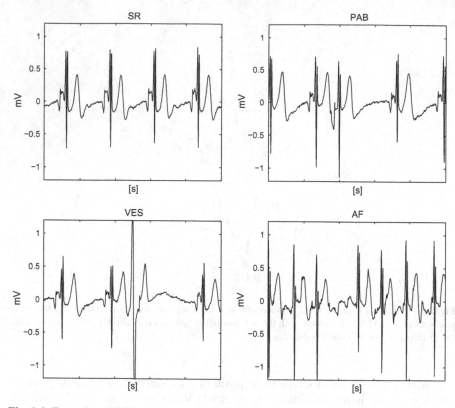

Fig. 1.6 Examples of ECGs with sinus rhythm (*above left*), premature atrial beat (*above right*), ventricular extra systole (*below left*) and atrial fibrillation (*below right*)

of the medical personnel in hospitals, health clinics, homes for the elderly and health resorts. Differential leads ECG sensors can either be used as a standalone devices to obtain one lead, or in tandems of three devices for the purpose of synthesizing 12-lead ECG (or some other lead system).

After the implementation of the above technical performances for an ECG body sensor, it is evident from Fig. 1.6 that the quality of the ECG signal is adequate for further clinical use. Four measurements from a single person are shown in this figure, obtained by measuring the potential difference between the standard positions of the leads V1 and V2, which was previously defined as a body sensor ECG. In order to show the real informational value of the measurements, the signals are presented in their raw form without filtering. A sinus rhythm (SR) and premature atrial beat (PAB) are shown above, on the left and the right, respectively. In the lower part of Fig. 1.6 examples of ventricular extra systole (VES) and atrial fibrillation (AF) are shown on the left and the right, respectively.

We can recognize all characteristic ECG waves (P, QRS, T) in the SR with similar time intervals between consecutive beats; arrhythmic beats PAB and VES have shapes and timings different from those of SR beats. In PAB, the P-wave is reversed, while in VES, the extra systole has no P-wave. However, the depolarization of the atria (P-wave) is visible near the beginning of the T-wave of the VES. The AF is characterized by the absence of P-wave, faster beat rate and unstructured consecutive beat intervals.

1.5 Book Summary by Chapters

The book topics are collected in chapters that can also be read independently. This chapter presents a short history of ECG evolution and lists crucial motivations and goals for the development of mHealth. Further, basic principles and facts related to electrocardiography are presented with a short description of the differential ECG that can be measured by a body sensor. The chapter concludes with this book summary by chapters.

A more detailed discussion in Chap. 2 aims to clarify the basic principles of multichannel electrocardiography and introduces the principle of differential ECG that enables an implementation of a small and unobtrusive wearable ECG sensor appropriate for long-term mobile health monitoring. It is shown how the sensor ECG could be used for heart rhythm analysis. The multi-functionality of the wearable sensor is addressed, which could implement the fusion of measurements of most important vital signs: ECG, respiration, activity, and others.

Design requirements of an evidence-based mHealth system and the functionality of a mobile application are presented in Chap. 3. The main difference between body ECG sensors and ambulatory ECG recorders is in the user interface. The smartphone makes for a great platform—it is becoming ubiquitous, it surpasses the required computing and communication capabilities, and provides the means of data analysis and exchange among stakeholders along the healthcare chain. The software on the smartphone can implement an interface that is already familiar to most users.

In Chap. 4, the visualization and analysis of the measured ECGs is addressed from the practical point of view. The described methodologies are tested in two ECG pilot systems. The first pilot is devoted to the analysis of atrial fibrillation in a seven day period after cardiac surgery. The second pilot is devoted to the screening of patients for irregular heartbeats in a healthcare center. The examination procedures that have to be done by medical practitioners are also presented.

Because the standard 12-lead ECG is still a golden standard in electrocardiography, Chap. 5 explains how the standard 12-lead ECG can be synthesized from a small number of differential leads. The explanation is supported by a theoretical background from lead theory with implications to the differential lead measurements interpretation and body sensor positioning.

Chapter 6 is a survey of existing related solutions based on wireless body ECG sensors. Most of the measurements shown in this book have been obtained by our laboratory prototypes of ECG body sensors and by its commercial version Savvy, which is also compared with other currently available ECG sensor-based solutions. Even though this chapter will become obsolete with time, it will give evidence about the initial attempts to establish an unobtrusive and economic mHealth system tailored to users, their caregivers and medical practitioners.

Chapter 7 provides a brief look on the near future mHealth capacity, based on the presented material and the current level of technological development. The main focuses of the discussion are technology, usability and potentially increased users' awareness for their own health. The book concludes with an overview of the presented topics and with a summary of expected benefits for users. Some comments about the future developments of mHealth systems are given. Finally, there is a list of relevant references and an index to the essential keywords used throughout the book.

References

1. Trobec, R.: Computer analysis of multichannel ECG. Comput. Biol. Med. **33**(3), 215–226 (2003)
2. Schiller, A.G.: Switzerland. Physician's Guide, ECG Measurements and Interpretation Programs (2009)
3. Zellerhoff, C., Himmrich, E., Nebeling, D., Przibille, O., Nowak, B., Liebrich, A.: How can we identify the best implantation site for an ECG event recorder? Pacing Clin. Electrophysiol. **23**, 1545–1549 (2000)
4. De Capua, C., Meduri, A., Morello, R.: A smart ECG measurement system based on web-service-oriented architecture for telemedicine applications. IEEE Trans. Instr. Meas. **59**(10), 2530–2538 (2010)
5. Bifulco, P., Cesarelli, M., Fratini, A., Ruffo, M., Pasquariello, G., Gargiulo, G.: A wearable device for recording of biopotentials and body movements. In: Proceedings of the IEEE International Workshop on Medical Measurements and Applications Proceedings (MeMeA), 2011, pp. 469–472
6. Pantelopoulos, A., Bourbakis, N.G.: A survey on wearable sensor-based systems for health monitoring and prognosis. IEEE Trans. Syst. Man Cybern.—Part C: Appl. Rev. **40**(1) (2010)
7. Lindén, M., Björkman, M.: Embedded sensor systems for health—providing the tools in future healthcare. Stud. Health Technol. Inf. **200**, 161–163 (2014)
8. P.W. Macfarlane, T.D.V. Lawrie (eds.): Comprehensive Electrocardiology, Theory and Practice in Health and Disease. Pergamon Press (1989)
9. Depolli, M., Avbelj, V., Trobec, R.: Computer-simulated alternative modes of U-wave genesis. J. Cardiovasc. Electrophysiol. **19**(1), 84–89 (2008)
10. Antzelevitch, C.: Cellular basis for the repolarization waves of the ECG. Ann. NY Acad. Sci. **2006**, 268–281 (1080)
11. Chikamori, T., Takata, J., Seo, H., Matsumura, Y., Kitaoka, H., Sugimoto, K., Doi, Y.: Diagnostic significance of an exercise-induced prominent U wave in acute myocardial infarction. Am. J. Cardiol. **78**(11), 1277–1281 (1996)

Chapter 2
From Multichannel ECG to Wireless Body Sensors

Abstract A more detailed description of multichannel electrocardiography and the differential lead aims to clarify why the multichannel ECG opens a path towards implementation of wireless wearable sensors. Several ways of how the differential lead could be used for heart rhythm monitoring are shown with options for analysis and interpretation of sensor ECG measurements. Finally, the most important vital signs that could be provided by a multifunctional body sensor are presented.

2.1 Multichannel ECG

The body potentials can be measured simultaneously in many positions on the body, e.g., up to 300, by a multichannel ECG. However, such devices have been regarded as non-practical for clinical use because of their complexity, related to the burden of connection wires and electrodes, and because of complex analysis of a huge amount of acquired ECG data. On the other hand, a single-channel body ECG sensor [1] still represents a viable solution for the detection of many cardiac problems, including arrhythmias and conduction abnormalities.

A path from a multichannel ECG to a multifunctional sensor is described in more detail in the rest of this chapter. The multichannel electrocardiography (MECG) is an extension of the conventional electrocardiography. It is aimed at refining the non-invasive characterization of cardiac activity. Increased spatial sampling on the body surface provides more information on potentials generated by the heart [2, 3]. An instructive method for representing MECG signals is the body surface mapping (BSM) [4]. Such a representation can be given with isocontours, e.g. isopotential contours, in which case the map shows the body surface potential at a specific moment, or isointegral contours, in which case the map shows the distribution of the sum of potentials over a specified time interval (QRS, ST 40, etc.), or similar.

Various MECG systems have been used for deriving BSMs, with the number of electrodes ranging from 10 to 300 [5, 6]. The result of an MECG measurement are time series of sampled body surface potential differences, encapsulating the data collected by all the electrodes at each sampling time. These potentials can be presented by a BSM that visualizes, by isocontours, the interpolated MECG measurements.

R. Trobec et al., *Body Sensors and Electrocardiography*, SpringerBriefs in Applied Sciences and Technology, DOI 10.1007/978-3-319-59340-1_2

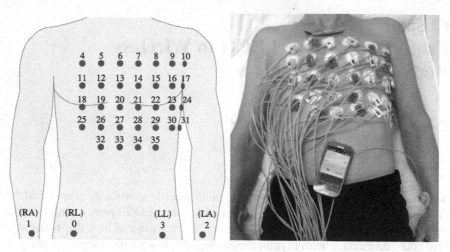

Fig. 2.1 Placing and numbering of 35 MECG electrodes (*left*) and an actual MECG system during a measurement with an ECG sensor in the top row (*right*)

The MECG measurements constitute a powerful research tool, because the redundant data can be used to validate findings, particularly in the cases when the interpretation of the conventional 12-lead ECG is not obvious. Such cases are, for example, when the signals from the electrodes are disturbed, or if the spatial variability of the heart parameters has to be examined [7, 8].

We have developed a custom-designed MECG device with 35 electrodes already in the 1990s [9] and have later acquired notable experiences with the acquisition of MECG measurements under different circumstances in laboratories and hospitals. The body potentials are measured as 32 unipolar leads referenced to the WCT, with electrodes placed on the thorax, and as standard 3 bipolar leads (I, II, III) with the electrodes placed on the limbs, i.e., one on each arm and one on the left leg. The right leg electrode (electrode 0) was also used for a ground reference. Equidistant positioning of the electrodes on the thorax is mostly used, but the MECG device allows also for a different positioning, if required. The equidistant positioning is often preferred because it enables simple BSM generation in which the measured potential differences from the electrodes are used directly, without a complicated weighted interpolation.

The preferred positioning and numbering of the 35 MECG electrodes is schematically shown in the left part of Fig. 2.1. The MECG system, during a measurement, is shown in the right part of Fig. 2.1. Note that an early prototype of the ECG sensor is connected in parallel with the MECG electrodes 5 and 7. The measured sensor ECG is shown on the smartphone. Further details on this particular MECG device can be found in [10].

As explained previously, the MECG measurements are values of local body surface potentials referenced to a selected reference point, e.g. the WCT, or alternatively the potential differences between two electrodes, e.g. standard bipolar leads, or also a

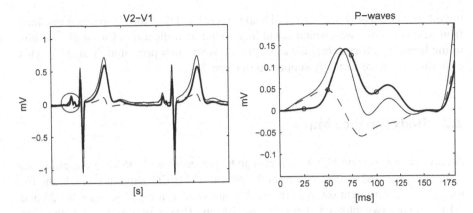

Fig. 2.2 Simultaneous measurements of the standard V1 (*dashed line*) and V2 (*solid line*) leads and the differential lead V2-V1 (*bold line*) for two consecutive beats (*left*), and a magnified PR interval of the first beat (*right*)

differential lead between two nearby MECG electrodes. An example of two MECG signals from the electrodes 12 and 14, and the differential lead signal from these electrodes, are shown in Fig. 2.2. Note that the MECG electrodes 12 and 14, as numbered in the left part of Fig. 2.1, can be used as an approximation of the standard leads V1 and V2. The signals shown in Fig. 2.2 were captured simultaneously with 1000 samples per second and filtered by a 50 Hz low-pass filter.

According to the explanation in Chap. 1 and Fig. 1.5, the difference V2-V1 is the differential lead or the ECG that can be measured by a body sensor with its electrodes positioned on the standard places of the V1 and V2 electrodes. The magnified PR interval from the first beat, marked with a circle in the left part of Fig. 2.2, is shown in the right part of Fig. 2.2. The P-wave was selected because its analysis is crucial for the study of the heart rhythm. The measurement confirms the high fidelity of the ECG. Note that the scale of the right graph is larger than the scale of the left graph for better reproduction of the P-waves morphology. The samples at 25, 50, 75 and 100 ms after the start of the atrial depolarization, i.e., the onset of the P wave, are marked with small circles.

It can be seen that the P wave in the differential lead has similar timing for both standard leads. As explained, the differential lead represents the difference V2-V1. Therefore, it indicates the local gradient of the potential field between the standard leads. Comparing the P wave signals of the V1 and V2 leads (thin curves) with the P wave signal from the differential lead (bold curve), several interesting facts can be noticed. The amplitude of the P wave signal from the differential lead at 25 ms is close to zero, because the leads V1 and V2 are on the same potential at these moments. The peak of the P wave from the differential lead near 75 ms is slightly shifted to the right, compared to the P wave from V2 lead, because of the negative potential at V1. The P wave from the differential lead at 100 ms is larger than the P waves from the V1 and V2 leads, again because of the negative signal on V1. We can suspect that the information from the differential lead is more local than the information obtained from the standard leads, which could help in the identification of local phenomena in the heart, e.g., focus areas for atrial [11] or ventricular premature beats [12]. This hypothesis is more formally supported in Chap. 5.

2.2 Body Surface Maps

An alternative view on MECG signals can be presented with BSMs. Four examples of isopotential BSMs, obtained from the presented MECG setup in Fig. 2.1, and for the same measurement setup as in Fig. 1.5, are shown in Fig. 2.3, again for 25 and 50 ms (upper two plots) and for 75 and 100 ms (lower two plots) after the start of atrial depolarization. The difference between two neighboring contours is 5 μV. The MECG electrode positions are marked with small circles. The ECG of the three missing MECG electrodes from the lowest horizontal line (in Fig. 2.1) have been extrapolated from signals of the neighboring electrodes, just to obtain a rectangular 7×5 grid. For example, the signal of the missing electrode in the position $(1,1)$ was obtained by averaging the signals of electrodes positioned in $(1,2)$ and $(2,1)$, which are numbered as 25 and 32, respectively. The approximated standard positions of V1 and V2, i.e. the MECG electrodes 12 and 14, are shown for comparison in the positions $(2,5)$ and $(4,5)$, respectively.

Since the differential lead is defined as a potential difference from two proximal points on the BSM, we can treat the measurement as a spatial derivative of the BSM, which can be obtained by the gradient of the measured MECG field of potentials:

$$\nabla BSM(x, y) = \frac{\partial BSM}{\partial x}\mathbf{i} + \frac{\partial BSM}{\partial y}\mathbf{j} \qquad (2.1)$$

where $\mathbf{i}$ and $\mathbf{j}$ are unit vectors in the x and y dimensions. The BSM gradient can be visualized by vectors that indicate the amount of the expected signal between two neighboring MECG electrodes, which is equivalent to the potential differences between the neighboring MECG electrodes. The gradients of the BSM potentials from Fig. 2.3 are shown in Fig. 2.4. This visualization can be used to help positioning the ECG sensor on an optimal place. A criterion for the selection of the best neighboring MECG electrodes that provide sufficient ECG signal could be the presence of large spatial derivatives throughout the PR interval. The component of the sum of vectors from Fig. 2.4, which is aligned with an imaginary straight line that connects both sensor electrodes, is the potential difference measured by the ECG sensor. We see that by this criterion, a good position is between the MECG electrodes 12 and 14, i.e., between the standard leads V1 and V2, which are also among the closest to the heart atria. There are also several other good positions, all in the vicinity of the heart.

Despite of their informative dominance, BSMs have not become a part of standard clinical procedures, because of the high complexity of MECG setup and because of

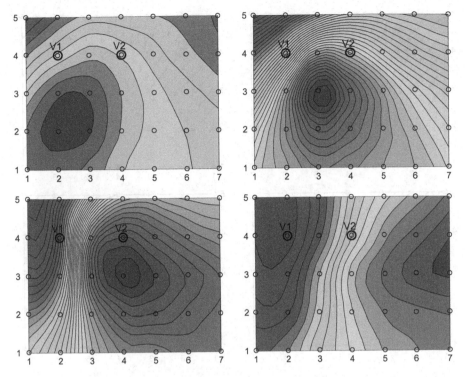

Fig. 2.3 Isopotential BSMs depicting the moments at 25 and 50 ms (*above*), and 75 and 100 ms (*below*), after the start of atrial depolarization

practical complications with many wired body electrodes. Furthermore, the interpretation of the BSM data is complex and still a part of ongoing research. However, in the era of high-performance ICT technologies and wireless communication, this situation may change if wireless and computerized MECG systems appear. In particular, a potential benefit from the analysis of BSM data is the provision of accurate methodologies for non-invasive analysis of the heart activity. With the advent of computers, powerful automatic algorithms can be implemented to process the measurements online, offering to medical practitioners more reliable and more specific diagnoses than the conventional 12-lead ECG.

From our early experience with the development of MECG systems and from MECG measurements, we have learned that the potential differences from closely positioned body electrodes provide a complete information about the heart rhythm. Furthermore, a "closer look" on the heart through the differential lead can elucidate more specific heart diagnoses. It is also evident that the signal-to-noise ratio decreases with the increase of the electrodes' proximity, which can result in lower accuracy of the measured ECG. Nevertheless, the breakthrough idea that enables the implementation of a small and wireless ECG sensor comes from our previous work in the area of MECG. We expect that in the near future, numerous online mHealth systems [13]

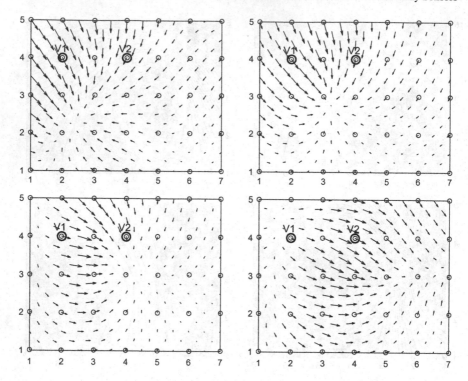

Fig. 2.4 Gradients of the isopotential BSMs from Fig. 2.3 at 25 and 50 ms (*above*), and 75 and 100 ms (*below*), after the start of atrial depolarization

will use a minimized set of sensors, with potentially personalized positioning, that will be able to synthesize the conventional 12-lead ECG. A more detailed discussion about this topic is given in Chap. 5.

2.3 Wireless Body Sensor

2.3.1 Prerequisites for Body Sensor Design

There are two major difficulties that have to be overcome to continuously and wirelessly measure electrical bio-potentials on a human body:

1. The bio-potentials reflect activities of living tissues, which are changing at intervals often much shorter than a single second. To get their reliable digital representation, the signals must usually be sampled more than hundred times per second. One has to either process the data measurements on the sensor or wirelessly transmit a large amount of streamed data to a more complex assisting device. In both

cases, a significant energy is consumed on the sensor because of the need for high computation or communication. Consequently, both implementation options limit the sensor autonomy. Usually, developers have to find an optimal combination between local computation and communication.

2. The electric potential differences cannot be measured between "wireless" points on the body; a conductive path (wire) is required between them for measuring the difference in the electric potential, i.e., the voltage. If the two connected points are close enough, they can be packed, together with the corresponding electronics, into a single body sensor.

A further goal of sensor developers has to be a technological solution for a medical grade multifunctional wireless body sensor with small dimensions (e.g., 10 cm) and a small weight (e.g., 15 g), which allows for unobtrusive use during every-day activities, exhaustive physical work, sleep and sports. The body sensor should be formatively designed so that it resembles an ornament, to make it more appealing to the users. However, it must also be fixed on the body reliably, and be taken on and off without damaging the skin. The distance between the electrodes should be small, but still sufficient to guarantee the signal-to-noise ratio required for accurate measurements. As said, the sensor should be multifunctional because users are ready to wear just a few sensors, ideally a single one, at a time. It should sense vital physiological signs (ECG, muscular activity, respiration, etc.) and relevant environmental parameters (acceleration, light intensity, temperature, etc.).

Finally, the body sensor should have a long autonomy, e.g., one week or more, a low-power wireless connection to a smartphone or some other personal assisting device, and should be accompanied with a simple software for the marking of cardiac-related events, for the generation of ECG reports, and for the visualization and interpretation of measurements. Regarding the medical grade, a moderate resolution of the ECG and eventual other signals should be suitable for long-term personal cardiac activity monitoring, as well as for clinical use. The fusion of the acquired data, physiological and environmental, should increase the interpretability of the measurements and allow for ambient intelligence. The sensor should support solutions to every-day problems of the medical personnel in hospitals, health clinics, homes for the elderly and health resorts.

As an example, a multifunctional body sensor prototype that fulfills most of the above listed design goals and requirements is shown in the left part of Fig. 2.5. Through co-design by engineers, patients and medical practitioners, the prototype has been upgraded into the near-to-market version shown in the right part of Fig. 2.5. Note that the body sensor is small, light and flexible, and therefore minimally obtrusive for the users.

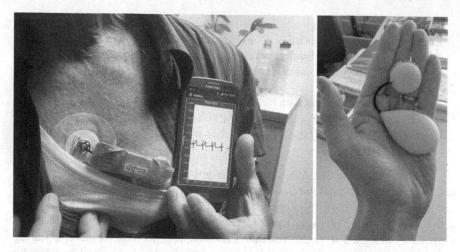

Fig. 2.5 An early prototype of an ECG body sensor connected through low-power Bluetooth with a mobile phone (*left*) and a near-to-market ECG sensor in a flexible design (*right*)

2.3.2 Positioning of an ECG Body Sensor

It can be expected that the body sensor ECG differs significantly in different positions. Some positions are better for monitoring atrial activities, particularly, morphologies of the P wave and types of arrhythmic events. The existing knowledge for the interpretation of the conventional 12-lead ECG is of limited use in the case of a wireless body sensor, because the latter neither has a fixed position nor is its output comparable with any standard lead. However, the existing knowledge is still useful for heart rhythm monitoring. Because the ECG body sensor gives a close look on the heart, it offers a novel type of electrocardiographic data that requires further research for proper interpretation [14].

Based on our experience from MECG measurements and on the investigation of BSMs and their gradients (see the explanation and Fig. 2.4 in the previous section), in the following, we propose some positions for the ECG body sensor, which give adequate results in the analysis of heart rhythm [15]. The positions are encoded with a simple labeling scheme shown in Fig. 2.6. Note that all positions are near the heart atrium to better capture the P wave. The reference point of the scheme is on the sternum, 5 cm superior to the xiphoid. To establish unambiguous labels of ECG sensor positions, four standard letters: L (left), R (right), S (superior) and I (inferior), are used. The first letter denotes the position of the positive electrode relative to the sternum, L or R. The positive electrode is located under the larger half of the sensor. We suppose that the sensor can be translated in steps of about 5 cm (or half of the sensor length) in the horizontal direction (towards L or R), which is denoted with the second letter. Any translation in the vertical direction, towards S or I, again

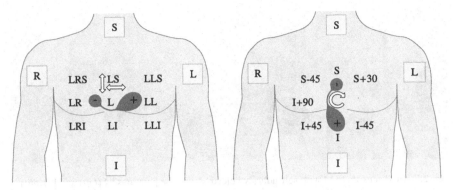

Fig. 2.6 Labeled positions of the sensor obtained by translation in a 5 cm mesh (*left*), and labeled positions of the sensor obtained by rotation for a selected angle in degrees (*right*)

for about 5 cm, is denoted with the third letter. Note that positions with nil or only one translation are labeled with less letters; e.g., position LL is at the level of the reference point, moved to the left for 5 cm.

The position of the sensor shown in the left part of Fig. 2.6 is labeled with L, because the larger half of the sensor (the positive electrode) is left from the sternum and the sensor center is above the reference point—no translation has been applied. The standard ECG leads V1 and V2 are 5 cm towards S, and the corresponding position of the ECG sensor that would be placed in the positions of the V1 and V2 electrodes is labeled with LS. If the sensor is moved from the reference point 5 cm towards I, the sensor position would be labeled with LI or LLI, if it is positioned more to the left. The sensor position above the right atrium and with the positive electrode directed to the left is labeled with LRS. By analogy, the initial L can be replaced with R, if the positive electrode of the ECG sensor is placed on the right side of the reference point, e.g., mirrored around the transfer axis. In this case, the measured signals are reversed in amplitudes if compared with the signals obtained in the positions labeled with the initial letter L.

Alternatively, the ECG sensor can be rotated around its center, in steps of about 45° with the clockwise direction (from the right to the left) regarded as the positive one. In these cases, the first letter, S or I, denotes the position of the positive electrode relative to the reference point. The second place in the label is reserved for the + or − sign and the angle in degrees, denoting the direction and the amount of rotation, e.g., I+45 or I−45, which means that the sensor is rotated from the vertical position with inferior positive electrode for 45° in the positive or in the negative direction, respectively. Again, the initial letter I can be replaced with S, which results in mirrored sensor positions. The labeled positions of the sensor obtained by rotation are shown in the right part of Fig. 2.6. The presented sensor position is labeled with I, because the positive electrode is below (inferior to) the reference point and no rotation has been applied.

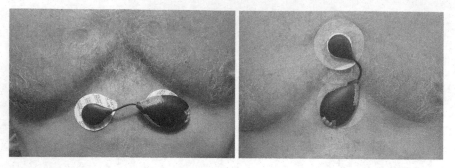

Fig. 2.7 ECG sensors fixed with self-adhesive electrodes in the positions LI (*left*) and I (*right*)

Two ECG sensors fixed with self-adhesive electrodes, at the often used positions labeled with LI and I, are shown in the left and the right part of Fig. 2.7, respectively.

Sometimes the ECG sensor cannot be positioned in any of the defined places, because of anatomical or other reasons, such as a surgery wound, furriness, etc. In such cases, one can use modified positions, labeled more precisely with additional letters and numbers. For example, if the ECG sensor is moved from the position I+45 towards the right for 5 cm, its label will be I+45R5, or if the ECG sensor is moved from the position LLS further to the left for 3 cm and up for 2 cm, its label will be LLSL3S2. Note that the rotation step could be also finer than 45°. Any additional characters, however, make the positioning labels more complex. Therefore, they will be used only in some special cases or when higher accuracy of the ECG sensor positioning is needed.

It is evident that the proposed notation results in several equivalent positions, such as L and S+90, or S-45 and I+135. There are also several mirrored positions, such as S and I, or S-45 and I-45, that just provide inverted signals and amplitudes. In any case, while the proposed labeling scheme can be useful in in-depth analysis of the heart rhythm, it can become too complicated for users. They most probably would prefer a short list of predefined, possibly graphically presented positions, from which they can choose before the measurement directly in the mobile application. In each of the presented measurements, we therefore inserted also a schematic graphical presentation of the ECG sensor position used for the particular measurements.

The ECG signal segments obtained when placing the ECG sensor in the nine positions from the left part of Fig. 2.6 are shown in Fig. 2.8. Note that all the signals are accurate enough for a reliable detection of all characteristic ECG waves, but the largest signals have been measured in the positions L, LRI and LI. The P wave is clearly visible in all positions except in LLS.

Figure 2.9 shows four ECGs recorded with the ECG sensor in the positions I+135, I+90, I+45 and I, as labeled in the right part of Fig. 2.6. Note that all four signals are accurate enough to determine all ECG waves and the heart rhythm. The signal from the position I+135 can be labeled also with S-45, which is an equivalent sensor position. The signal from the position I+90 is in fact the inverted signal from the mirror position L, and can also be labeled with R.

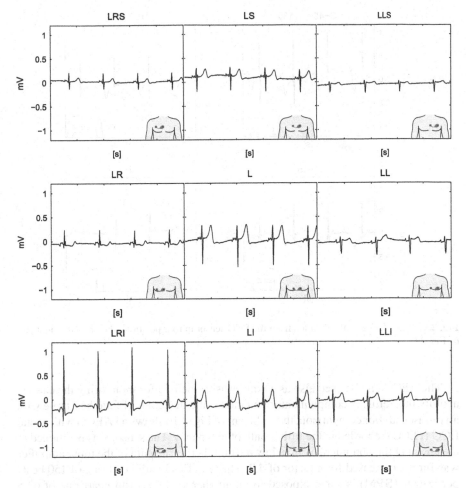

Fig. 2.8 Raw ECG signals obtained from the ECG sensor in the positions shown in the left part of Fig. 2.6

The sensitivity of the ECG body sensor is demonstrated with the recorded abdominal ECG (AECG) in Fig. 2.10. Note that the scale of the graphs is increased because of small signals. The AECG in the left part of Fig. 2.10 was recorded with the ECG sensor placed on the left part of the abdomen at the level of the umbilicus of the same person as in the recordings in Figs. 2.8 and 2.9. Note that the amplitude of the AECG signal is about 0.2 mV, which is significantly smaller than in the previous examples. Therefore, the recording can only suffice for the detection of the heart rate.

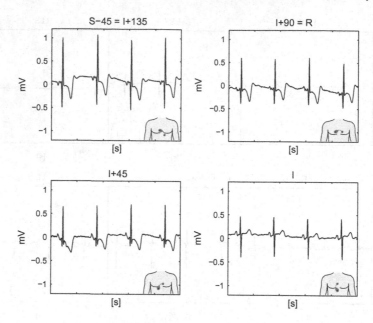

Fig. 2.9 Raw ECG signals obtained from the ECG sensor in four positions shown in the right part of Fig. 2.6

The AECG can be used also as a non-invasive method for monitoring the cardiac activity of a fetus. A complementary method is the detection of fetal heart rate with an ultrasound. For comparison, the right part of Fig. 2.10 shows an AECG with a fetal ECG (FECG) recorded in the fifth month of pregnancy. The sensor was positioned in the center of the abdomen, 5 cm below the umbilicus. The gain of the input amplifier was further increased for a factor of 4.7. The fetal ECG with heart rate of 150 beats per minute (BPM) is superimposed to the mother's AECG with heart rate of 62.5 BPM. Since the fetus is very small, its ECG signal measured on the abdomen during pregnancy has an extremely small amplitude, significantly smaller than the amplitude of the mother's AECG. Therefore, the scale of the graph is further increased. Note that in the fifth month of pregnancy, the size of the fetus' left heart ventricle is only about 15 mm [16]. The AECG peak-to-peak QRS amplitude is approximately 40 μV, while the QRS amplitude of the FECG is about 15 μV. The recordings demonstrate the remarkable potential of the ECG body sensor for AECG measurements. The interference from the power grid is not present in the signal, which is crucial for further analysis.

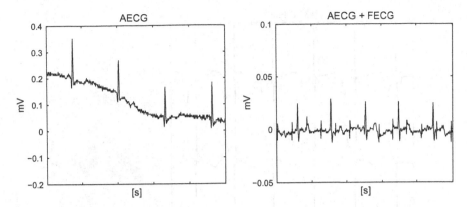

Fig. 2.10 Raw AECG signal obtained with the ECG sensor positioned on the left part of the abdomen at the level of the umbilicus (*left*), and AECG recorded in the fifth month of pregnancy with the sensor positioned in the center of the abdomen, 5 cm below the umbilicus (*right*)

2.3.3 Multiple Body Sensors

So far we have demonstrated the use of a single ECG sensor placed on different locations in the vicinity of the heart. To acquire more information, two sensors, each in a different position, can be used for simultaneous measurement of ECG. Such an approach could be beneficial for better detection of the propagation direction of depolarization waves and consequently for detailed study of the excitation areas. However, new knowledge is needed for proper interpretation of such ECG measurements.

As an example, two concurrently measured ECGs from two independent sensors are shown in the left part of Fig. 2.11. For easier comparison, the measured ECG signals are shown in two graphs vertically separated by 1 mV. The upper graph was obtained from the ECG sensor in the position I+30, while the lower graph from the position I-30. The actual positions of both sensors are shown on the photo in the right part of Fig. 2.11. We see that the morphology of the P waves has changed after the third beat, which could indicate a shift between two atrial excitation focuses. Based on the signals and the knowledge about sensors' positions, an expert electro physiologist could determine the paths of depolarization fronts and consequently the locations of both focuses.

If we further increase the number of sensors, e.g. to three, and place them on appropriate positions, the acquired information can be used for an accurate synthesis of the standard 12-lead ECG. This important topic is described in more detail in Chap. 5.

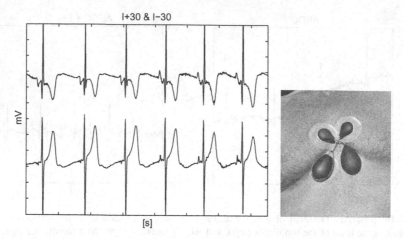

Fig. 2.11 Concurrent measurements from two sensors in the positions I+30 (*graph above*) and I-30 (*graph below*) are shown on the *left*; a photo of the ECG sensors fixed on the body is shown on the *right*

2.4 Multi-functionality of Body Sensors

Hand watches could be historically regarded as the earliest wearable sensors, because they originally provided the timekeeping function. Today, smart watches are available, equipped with sensors able to measure vital signs and with a miniature computer that can analyze the acquired data and communicate with the users and their social networks. The classic hand watches have become so popular because of the beneficial data which they provide, because of their personalized formative design and because of their simple usage, in spite of the complicated mechanism inside. The habit of wearing two hand watches simultaneously, however, has never become popular. It seems that most users, if not seriously stimulated by urgent needs, are ready to wear just a single sensor.

Regarding ECG body sensors, the following aspects have to be considered. The first aspect, related to the implementation of ECG body sensors, is the proximity of the two electrodes that aim to measure a body surface potential difference, which can be measured only if both body electrodes are electrically connected with a data acquisition system. The proximity of the electrodes is important in the context of body sensors because the users have to consider both electrodes as a single wearable unit.

The next aspect, related to the mobility and non-obtrusive use, is the ability of wearable sensors to act as wireless units, which substantially improves their usability and acceptability by the users. However, a lot of work remains to be done in order to select the correct balance between the complexity of the communication protocols, the ability for local signal processing, memory requirements, and the power consumption related to the autonomy of the sensor.

Finally, from the aspect of multi-functionality, sensors that measure the ECG potential difference on the body surface should also provide information on other vital functions, either directly (e.g., for muscular activity, skin resistance, movement, skin temperature, humidity and light) or indirectly (e.g., for respiration), by a customized analysis of the ECG signal. The following subsections present some initial results supporting the proposed multi-functionality approach and the fusion of the measured data for more reliable diagnoses.

2.4.1 Muscular Activity

Surface electromyography (sEMG) is an established non-invasive method for assessing the skeletal muscular activity. If the sensor is placed in the vicinity of the heart, the sEMG signal is superimposed on the ECG and is usually regarded as an unwanted signal disturbance. This is usually the case when one is primarily interested in measuring the heart activity. If the sensor is placed on a specific muscle, however, it can act as a regular sEMG sensor. By using the sensor measurements as an input to a dedicated software, specific muscular activity could be detected and interpreted.

We have performed an experiment where the ECG sensor was placed on the right-hand biceps brachii muscle of a male subject, following the SENIAM recommendations [17] (see left part of Fig. 2.12). A measuring protocol, based on the variation of the time intervals and the muscular load, is presented in Table 2.1.

The corresponding rectified sEMG signal (in blue), sampled at 125 Hz, with marked intervals defined by the measurement protocol from Table 2.1, is shown in the right part of Fig. 2.12. The red graph is the amplitude envelope estimated by the "EMG amplitude estimation toolbox" described in [18]. This toolbox implements a six-stage algorithm for sEMG amplitude estimation: noise filtering, whitening, multiple-channel combination, demodulation, smoothing and re-linearization. From Fig. 2.12, it is clearly visible that high amplitudes of the measured sEMG correlate well with high muscular loads.

Table 2.1 Muscular activity—sEMG measurement protocol

Interval name	Duration (s)	Description
none	0–30	Movement of fingers
a	30–40	Fast lift of 4 kg weight
b	40–65	Slow lift and hold of 4 kg weight
c	65–80	Slow lift and hold of 6 kg weight
d	80–90	Slow lift and hold of 6 kg weight
e	90–110	Two slow lifts of 12 kg weight

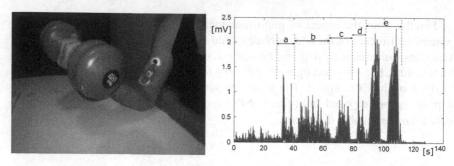

Fig. 2.12 Experimental setup for recording biceps brachii sEMG (*left*). The sEMG measurement obtained in the experiment defined in Table 2.1 (*right*)

One possible application of the sEMG obtained by a wireless ECG body sensor is in physiotherapy. A muscle activation is monitored using sEMG, so that users percept auditory or visual stimulus for their activity (biofeedback). Another application is in the monitoring of sport activities. The obtained sEMGs can be used to assess the force generated by a muscle [19] or the amount of fatigue in a muscle [20]. Additionally, the sEMG obtained by an ECG sensor can be used in combination with other sensors, such as accelerometers, for monitoring the physical activity of specific professionals (occupational bio-mechanics), or for remote exercise monitoring.

An additional potential benefit from sEMG is the ability to detect muscular activities for purposes other than body movement. For example, the breathing rate can be extracted to some extent from a recorded ECG, which is evident from the 20 seconds of raw ECG measurement shown in Fig. 2.13. For this particular measurement, the ECG sensor was placed in the position LI (see Fig. 2.6). The sEMG signal is visible as a low-amplitude noise, superimposed over the ECG signal during four deep inhales. Note that the variation in the ECG amplitude is in a close correlation with the

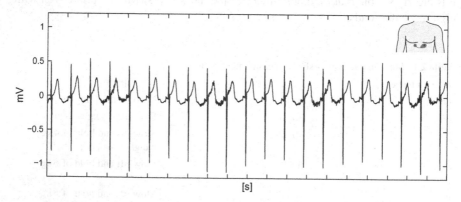

Fig. 2.13 A 20 s ECG sensor measurement with a "noise" from the muscular activity during four respiration cycles

sEMG. Such additional information about the respiration could contribute, in combination with other methods, for reliable detection of the respiration rate. The observed amplitude variation is the basis for the technique of ECG-derived respiration, which is described in the next subsection.

2.4.2 Respiration Derived from ECG

Breathing is one of the most characteristic vital signs and can reflect the status of a patient or the progression of an illness. The cyclic process that starts with inhale and ends with exhale is referred to as breathing or respiration cycle. The respiratory rate indicates the frequency of breathing and can be obtained from the time between two consecutive inhales or exhales. Any deviations in the respiratory rate can help predict potentially serious clinical events, such as a cardiac arrest, or may suggest that a patient has to be admitted to an intensive-care unit [21].

ECG-derived respiration (EDR) techniques [22] are based on two observations. First, the ECG electrodes fixed on the chest move relative to the heart. Second, the transthoracic impedance varies as the lungs fill and empty. Both phenomena influence the amplitude of the recorded ECG and thus a careful analysis of an ECG can be used to derive the breathing rate. Another well-known method of breathing rate derivation is based on the knowledge that the beat-to-beat interval varies primarily due to respiratory sinus arrhythmia (RSA). The heart rate variability (HRV) induced by RSA is more pronounced in young and healthy subjects, which is one of the limitations of this method [23] when applied on older subjects.

In the review paper [24], electrical impedance pneumography across the chest and a photoplethysmogram of a finger were fused to achieve very robust results. The estimation of the breathing rate was still limited by artefacts introduced by movements. Thirteen different algorithms for the detection of sleep apnoea from ECG recordings were analyzed in [25]. The algorithms were based on the frequency-domain features to estimate the changes in the heart rate and the respiration rate. The respiration-related HRV is reduced in the elderly, but the ECG waveform amplitude variability persists regardless of age. Hence, the latter approach could provide better overall performance.

All the above-mentioned approaches for breathing rate derivation are based on wired electrodes and external devices that cannot be considered as a body sensor. It can be expected that the ECG body sensor, placed on the chest near the heart, can reliably estimate the respiration rate by analyzing the QRS amplitudes. The results could be further improved by concurrent measurement of the impedance between the two electrodes.

A simple algorithm for the derivation of the respiration rate can be designed from the following functional blocks: QRS detection, baseline wandering removal, interpolation of QRS amplitudes to obtain the envelope of the respiration-induced variations, resampling of the interpolated QRS amplitudes. The final phase of the algorithm is the detection of the respiration cycles from the re-sampled QRS ampli-

Fig. 2.14 ECG measured with an ECG body sensor (*red graph*) and respiration measured with a thermistor (*gray graph*). All 58 R- and S-peaks (*blue points*) and 11 respiration cycles (*blue circles*) have been correctly detected

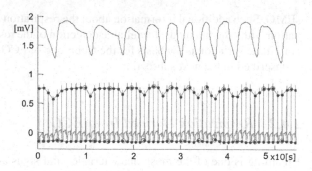

tudes variations induced by respiration. QRS and respiration cycles can be detected relatively simply, because of their characteristic periodic variations in amplitudes, which makes this method relatively easy to implement.

An algorithm that can reliably extract respiration rates from variations in the R-peak amplitudes is described and evaluated in more detail in [26]. The principal approach is visualized in Fig. 2.14. The ECG measurement of 53 seconds (red graph) was obtained from a ECG body sensor in the position I according to the notation in Fig. 2.6. At the same time, for validation of the EDR algorithm, the temperature of the inhaled and exhaled air (gray graph) was measured at the nasal exit.

We see that all 58 R-peaks and 58 S-peaks (blue points) have been correctly detected by a QRS detector. By comparing the amplitude of the R-peaks (blue graph) with the temperature of the respiration air, we can see a strong correlation. Eleven respiration cycles are clearly visible as changes of the R-peak amplitudes. However, a false positive respiration cycle nine was identified in the R-peaks variations. Still, a run of the same algorithm on the S-peaks correctly detected all eleven respiration cycles.

A more extensive study published in [26] has identified several sensor positions near the center of the chest which provide good ECG signals for the EDR technique. However, most of the positions shown in Fig. 2.6 can also be used for EDR, which confirms that the measurements from a single ECG body sensor can provide two seemingly independent measurements, i.e., the heart rate and the respiration rate.

2.4.3   Activity Detection

Movements and other activities can be monitored by solid-state inertial sensors, e.g., a 6-degrees-of-freedom unit with 3-axis accelerometer for measuring translation and 3-axis gyroscopes for measuring rotations. Such units are implemented as miniature micro-electro-mechanical systems (MEMS) and can be easily incorporated into the basic wireless ECG body sensor. The sampling rate of an activity sensor depends on the application, but for simple detection of user's movements, which are mostly of a low frequency, it can be kept low to limit the power consumption. Alternatively, the analysis of activity sensor measurements can be done locally on the sensor and only predefined features, which have reached the specified threshold values, are transmitted over a radio link. When the user is at rest, only Earth's gravity is measured, which can provide information about the sensor's orientation. By a concurrent analysis of ECG and acceleration, a more in-depth and robust analysis of vital functions can be made, which allows for generating also reliable alerts of dangerous states. For example, the maximal heart rate in resting should not be higher than 100 BPM, while during an intensive physical activity it can be as high as 180 BPM or even more. Also, the heart rate cannot increase momentarily and significantly if the user is not active. A potential reason for such an event could be in an emotional stress or a tachyarrhythmia.

We know that an optimal position of the ECG sensor is in the vicinity of the heart, which is not ideal for the classification of all user's movements, but is still acceptable for activity detection [27]. By using a more complex and real-time data analysis on the inertial data, the recognition of the user's activities and detection of falls can be implemented. Simpler data analysis algorithms are based on predictable and robust rules that help to recognize the static states. Machine-learning based classifiers can further recognize movements, e.g. a fall or a jump, for which the rules alone are not sufficient.

Compared to the previously listed applications, where EMG and QRS amplitude variations are superimposed to the ECG sensor signal, reliable activity recognition requires two independent measurements from two inertial sensors, placed in different positions on the body [27]. Because the measurements are performed with separate sensors with asynchronous clocks, an important additional task appears in data analysis, i.e., synchronization of data streams. The synchronization can be accomplished by the analysis of timestamps inserted into the measurement stream at the time of data sampling [28]. The synchronized signals are then segmented and forwarded to the analysis pipeline that is split in two paths. In one path, the segmented data are transformed into feature vectors for the activity recognition module. In the other path, the fall detection module analyzes the accelerator signals for falls. For real-time analysis, the procedures are repeated several times per second, analyzing the last two seconds of the inertial signals. Further details about the algorithm implementation can be found in [29].

2.4.4 Data Fusion for More reliable diagnoses

In the previous sections, we described the design and development route of a wireless bipolar ECG body sensor for long-term monitoring of users' health status. Taking users' feedback into account, e.g. the notion of unobtrusiveness, and respecting the technical limitations, e.g. power autonomy and signal-to-noise ratio, one can develop a small body device able to measure multiple vital and environmental signals.

Based on our previous research, experimental work, feedback from users and medical practitioners, we propose what is in our opinion the optimal solution for mHealth-based long-term monitoring of vital signals:

- Data acquisition should be performed by a single wireless body device comprising of several sensors and thus able to measure several physiological and physical quantities.
- Multiple parameters should be extracted from a single data source whenever possible, e.g., respiration and EMG from the ECG data.
- The sensor should be able to function autonomously for several days, preferably weeks.
- Measurements should not be required to be strictly continuous—their value lies in their long-term character. The users should be able to put the sensor down or wear it only when they feel comfortable wearing it. Likewise, the software for data analysis should be able to gracefully deal with intervals of missing data.
- Sensors should be used for further evidence-based medicine in areas of heart monitoring and diagnostics, optimization of medicament dosage, self-management of health and similar.

An mHealth system based on multi-functional sensors is able to provide complex real-time data streams, composed of fused data that can be efficiently analyzed by advanced data mining and machine-learning algorithms. The main goal behind the data fusion [30] is the ability of making more reliable alerts or diagnoses [31]. However, to be able to efficiently and reliably implement a complex data analytics on fused data, and to evaluate the required storage and computational resources, several aspects should be addressed.

Data synchronization: The streams of measured data are in general not aligned in time, but for data fusion, they should be synchronized. For example, the ECG and acceleration are obtained from independent sensors, which may run at different clocks or have own local analogue-to-digital converters, and are therefore inherently asynchronous. On the other hand, the signals derived from ECG and are superimposed to it are inherently synchronous with the ECG. The wireless transmission is the next step where the synchronization can deteriorate. The sensor data are transferred in consecutive packets, of which some could be—depending on the communication protocol—lost or delayed, e.g. because of network congestion. Several approaches to maintain the synchronism of data are known [32]. We implemented a simple one based on timestamps inserted into each data packet [28]. At the receiver side, based on the known sampling rate determined on the sensor side, the packets are analyzed and the real-time data is reconstructed. In the case of multiple ECG sensors with slightly different sampling clocks, the synchronization between the sensors is maintained on the basis of common events, e.g. R peaks in the ECG signal. Details about the clock synchronization are given in Sect. 2.3.

Communication and storage complexity: The current technological level of low-power radio communication can manage a low-range wireless transmission of data in the range of 10^4 bits/second, which is enough to cover the data transmission between the wireless body sensor and a smartphone. The data are collected in the smartphone and can eventually be forwarded to a computer Cloud for storage and further analysis, using more powerful existing mobile network infrastructure with no serious restrictions regarding the power consumption. Still, a problem of network congestion can arise in some cases, because of a huge amount of streamed and near real-time data. The accumulated measured ECG data can reach over 10^7 bytes/day, or approximately 0.5 GB/month/user, which is manageable by the current storage technology, even for several thousands of concurrent users and including measures necessary for medical-grade data reliability. The storage of long-term sensor data could be ultimately implemented in a distributed Cloud-based storage system.

Computational complexity: The program code of the data analytics algorithms should run in ultimate mHealth solutions on the local processor in the sensor, on the smartphone, and on a dedicated server or a computer in the Cloud. To be able to manage the response time of the visualization and analytic software in a reasonable frame, possibly in real time, the number of floating point operations per second (FLOPS) must remain proportional to the number of data samples, which could reach 10^4 bytes/second of fused data from a multifunctional body sensor. Assuming that 100 FLOPS are needed for an analysis of each byte, the computational complexity of data visualization and analytics results in 10^6 FLOPS. Additional computing resources are needed for data compression and encryption, which could contribute additional 100 FLOPS/byte. The estimated computational complexity per user is $2x10^6$ FLOPS or 2 MFLOPS. It can be further assumed that several phases of data analytics will be implemented on different processors (sensor, smartphone, monitoring center, Cloud) and that each user is equipped with a sensor and a smartphone, with independent measurements and computation that can run concurrently and in parallel. Assuming finally that a contemporary high-performance computer can manage around 50 GFLOPS, it follows that several ten thousands of users' data streams, e.g. 25.000, could be managed by a single dedicated high-performance computer. However, in reality, an overhead will be present, because of input/output data transfer within the computer. Therefore, it seems that a more reasonable estimation is several thousands of users. A bottleneck will certainly remain the assistance of medical experts who must confirm the diagnoses or alerts for each individual user. Further details about software implementation issues are given in the next section.

References

1. Trobec, R., Avbelj, V., Rashkovska, A.: Multi-functionality of wireless body sensors. The IPSI BgD Trans. Internet Res. **10**, 23–27 (2014)
2. Trobec, R.: Computer analysis of multichannel ECG. Comput. Biol. Med. **33**(3), 215–226 (2003)
3. Avbelj, V., Trobec, R., Gersak, B.: Beat-to-beat repolarisation variability in body surface electrocardiograms. Med. Biol. Eng. Comput. **41**(5), 556–560 (2003)

4. De Ambroggi, L., Musso, E., Taccardi, B.: Body surface mapping. In: Macfarlane, P.W., Lawrie, T.D.V. (eds.) Comprehensive Electrocardiology, Theory and Practice in Health and Disease. Pergamon Press (1989)
5. Lux, R.L., Smith, C.R., Wyatt, R.F., Abildskov, J.A.: Limited lead selection for estimation of body surface potential maps in electrocardiography. IEEE Trans. Biomed. Eng. 25(3), 270–276 (1978)
6. Gerstenfeld, E.P., SippensGroenewegen, A., Lux, R.L., Lesh, M.D.: Derivation of an optimal lead set for measuring ectopic atrial activation from the pulmonary veins by using body surface mapping. J. Electrocardiol. 33(Suppl), 179–185 (2000)
7. Yamada, T., Fukunami, M., Shimonagata, T., Kumagai, K., Sanada, S., Ogita, H., Asano, Y., Hori, M., Hoki, N.: Dispersion of signal-averaged p wave duration on precordial body surface in patients with paroxysmal atrial fibrillation. Eur. Heart J. 20(3), 211–220 (1999)
8. Gersak, B., Trobec, R., Gabrijelcic, T., Avbelj, V.: Comparison of the ST-40ms isointegral maps prior to and after aortocoronary revascularisation. Comput. Cardiol. 24, 505–507 (1997)
9. Avbelj, V.: Analiza električne aktivnosti srca s pomočjo večkanalne elektrokardiografije [Analysis of the heart's electrical activity by multichannel electrocardiography]. (Doctoral dissertation in Slovene language), Ph.D. thesis, University of Ljubljana, Slovenia (2003)
10. Avbelj, V., Trobec, R., Gersak, B., Vokac, D.: Multichannel ECG measurement system. In: Proceedings of the Tenth IEEE Symposium on Computer-Based Medical Systems, 1997, pp. 81–84
11. Boineau, J.P., Canavan, T.E., Schuessler, R.B., Cain, M.E., Corr, P.B., Cox, J.L.: Demonstration of a widely distributed atrial pacemaker complex in the human heart. Circulation 77(6), 1221–1237 (1988)
12. Ferrer, A., Sebastián, R., Sánchez-Quintana, D., Rodrìguez, J.F., Godoy, E.J., Martìnez, L., Saiz, J.: Detailed anatomical and electrophysiological models of human Atria and Torso for the simulation of atrial activation. PLOS ONE, 1–29 (2015)
13. Gorjup, V., Jazbec, A., Geršak, B.: Transtelephonic transmission of electrocardiograms in Slovenia. J. Telemed. Telecare 6(4), 205–208 (2000)
14. Hansen, I.H., Hoppe, K., Gjerde, A., Kanters, J.K., Sorensen, H.B.D.: Comparing twelve-lead electrocardiography with close-to-heart patch based electrocardiography. In: Proceedings of the 37th Annual International Conference of the IEEE Engineering in Medicine and Biology Society (EMBC), 2015, pp. 330–333
15. Puurtinen, M., Viik, J., Hyttinen, J.: Best electrode locations for a small bipolar ECG device: signal strength analysis of clinical data. Ann. Biomed. Eng. 37(2), 331–336 (2009)
16. Sharland, G., Allan, L.: Normal fetal cardiac measurements derived by cross-sectional echocardiography. Ultrasound Obstetr. Gynecol. 2(3), 175–181 (1992)
17. Hermens, H.J., Freriks, B., Disselhorst-Klug, C., Rau, G.: Development of recommendations for SEMG sensors and sensor placement procedures. J. Electromyogr. Kinesiol. 10(5), 361–374 (2000)
18. Clancy, E.A., Morin, E.L., Merletti, R.: Sampling, noise-reduction and amplitude estimation issues in surface electromyography. J. Electromyogr. Kinesiol. 12(1), 1–16 (2002)
19. Disselhorst-Klug, C., Schmitz-Rode, T., Rau, G.: Surface electromyography and muscle force: limits in sEMG-force relationship and new approaches for applications. Clin. Biomech. (Bristol, Avon) 24(3), 225–235 (2009)
20. Cifrek, M., Medved, V., Tonković, S., Ostojić, S.: Surface EMG based muscle fatigue evaluation in biomechanics. Clin. Biomech. (Bristol, Avon) 24(4), 327–340 (2009)
21. Cretikos, M.A., Bellomo, R., Hillman, K., Chen, J., Finfer, S., Flabouris, A.: Respiratory rate: the neglected vital sign. Med. J. Aust. 188(11), 657–659 (2008)
22. Al-Khalidi, F.Q., Saatchi, R., Burke, D., Elphick, H., Tan, S.: Respiration rate monitoring methods: a review. Pediatr. Pulmonol. 46(6), 523–529 (2011)
23. Langley, P., Bowers, E.J., Murray, A.: Principal component analysis as a tool for analyzing beat-to-beat changes in ECG features: application to ECG-derived respiration. IEEE Trans. Biomed. Eng. 57(4), 821–829 (2010)

24. Tarassenko, L., Mason, L., Townsend, N.: Multi-sensor fusion for robust computation of breathing rate. Electron. Lett. **38**, 1314–1316 (2002)
25. Penzel, T., McNames, J., Murray, A., de Chazal, P., Moody, G., Raymond, B.: Systematic comparison of different algorithms for apnoea detection based on electrocardiogram recordings. Med. Biol. Eng. Comput. **40**(4), 402–407 (2002)
26. Trobec, R., Rashkovska, A., Avbelj, V.: Two proximal skin electrodes-a respiration rate body sensor. Sensors (Basel) **12**(10), 13813–13828 (2012)
27. Gjoreski, H., Lustrek, M., Gams, M.: Accelerometer placement for posture recognition and fall detection. In: 7th International Conference on Intelligent Environments (IE), 2011, pp. 47–54
28. Trobec, R., Depolli, M., Avbelj, V.: Wireless network of bipolar body electrodes. In: Seventh International Conference on Wireless On-demand Network Systems and Services (WONS) (2010), pp. 145–150
29. Gjoreski, H., Rashkovska, A., Kozina, S., Luštrek, M., Gams, M.: Telehealth using ECG sensor and accelerometer. In: 37th International Convention on Information and Communication Technology, MIPRO (2014), pp. 270–274
30. Pantelopoulos, A., Bourbakis, N.: SPN-model based simulation of a wearable health monitoring system. Conf. Proc. IEEE Eng. Med. Biol. Soc. **2009**, 320–323 (2009)
31. Wilson, S.J., Wong, D., Pullinger, R.M., Way, R., Clifton, D.A., Tarassenko, L.: Analysis of a data-fusion system for continuous vital sign monitoring in an emergency department. Eur. J. Emerg. Med. **23**(1), 28–32 (2016)
32. Rhee, I.-K., Lee, J., Kim, J., Serpedin, E., Wu, Y.-C.: Clock synchronization in wireless sensor networks: an overview. Sensors (Basel) **9**(1), 56–85 (2009)

Chapter 3
Software for an mHealth System

Abstract A description of software requirements for an mHealth system is provided. Several layers of software are required for proper system functioning: ECG body sensor firmware, applications on smartphones, Cloud applications, and standalone applications for personal computers. The main functionality requirements of the mHealth software are described. Additionally, approaches for fulfilling those requirements are proposed.

3.1 Hardware Infrastructure

An mHealth system is powered by a complex ICT system and comprised of heavily inter-dependent functional modules. First of all, an mHealth system requires a device with computing, storage and interconnection capabilities, which the user can carry around at all times. So-called smart devices, such as tablets, smart watches and the ubiquitous smartphones, can readily fulfill this role [1]. From here on, we shall refer to smartphones only, because currently they are leaders among personal assistant devices. In the future, smart devices of some alternative form could take over this role.

Second, a sensing device that can measure one or more parameters related to the user's well-being is required. Smartphones could be used also for this purpose, but the system becomes far more efficient if it relies on dedicated sensing devices. A dedicated device can be tailored in design for accurate measurements of specific parameters. For medical-grade ECG measurements, for example, constant electrical contact of the measuring device with the chest is required.

A diagram of an mHealth system for ECG monitoring is given in Fig. 3.1. The figure depicts the user's view of the relevant ICT parts of the mHealth platform and the communication between them. The central component of the system is the user, interacting with the remaining components through a smartphone, a personal computer (optional) and an ECG body sensor. The role of the remaining components

© The Author(s) 2018
R. Trobec et al., *Body Sensors and Electrocardiography*, SpringerBriefs
in Applied Sciences and Technology, DOI 10.1007/978-3-319-59340-1_3

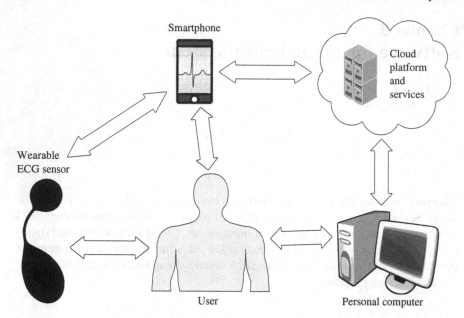

Fig. 3.1 The ICT components in an mHealth system from the user's point of view. The user interacts with an ECG body sensor, a smartphone and a personal computer, while Cloud services take care of data storage and processing. The smartphone acts as a hub for transferring data from the ECG body sensor to the Cloud. The smartphone and the personal computer both serve as an interface towards data stored on the Cloud

is twofold: to support the user in proactive health management and to collect data for analysis by medical practitioners. The ECG body sensor is used for sensing, that is, for measuring ECG, and for providing ambient and contextual information about the measurement. The ambient and contextual information can additionally be used to help in the analysis of the acquired ECG measurements. The user's interaction with the ECG body sensor is very limited—the user only wears the device. The smartphone is used for additional sensing, processing, interfacing with the ECG body sensor, visualization and alerting. It is the primary interface of the user towards the rest of the mHealth system. A personal computer would be used if the user wishes to analyze the acquired measurements beyond the scope of the real-time analysis provided by the smartphone. The Cloud platform represents the data link between the smartphone and the personal computer, and adds additional processing power, storage options and means of communication between the user and medical practitioners. The Cloud platform also enables access to the measured to the medical practitioners for diagnostic purposes.

3.2 Software

Several layers of software are required for proper system functioning. A coarse-grain division of the software into parts, according to where these parts are executed, is given below.

- *Custom software, also termed firmware, on the micro-controller-based sensing device.* The firmware controls data sampling and the storage, the analysis and the wireless transmission of sensor data to other modules.
- *An application on the smartphone.* The smartphone application acts as an interface between the mHealth system and its users, providing a convenient way for interaction with the sensing device. From the user's point of view, the application represents the core of the mHealth system. Thus, a user-friendly application design should be seen as one of the most important goals in the implementation of an mHealth system.
- *Cloud services implemented on the top of a Cloud platform.* Cloud services are already an established technical solution for data storage and analysis. They can provide custom views on the online measured health data for medical practitioners, for the users of the system, and potentially also for their caregivers. These services can also be seamlessly connected to the patient's electronic health records, which is crucial for making personalized diagnoses.
- *A set of computer programs that run on personal computers or mobile devices, able to process and visualize measurements off-line.* These applications represent an access interface to the Cloud services for medical practitioners and additional means of interaction with the mHealth system for its users. They could be built on the existing software used by the medical practitioners, by extending it with a module for accessing the Cloud services of the mHealth service. New software, which would be adapted to the type of the measurements gathered by the mHealth system, could also be developed. An example of an existing software suit that was modified to support measurements obtained from an mHealth system is described in Sect. 6.2.1.

3.3 mHealth Requirements

The main difference between mHealth and classical state-of-the-art ambulatory ECG recorders is in the user interface. A novel interface towards the user can transform an ambulatory recorder from a burden to an indispensable equipment for every-day life. On the other hand, the smartphone makes for a great platform for an mHealth system—it has become almost ubiquitous, it offers ample computing capabilities, and it provides means for communicating data along healthcare pathways.

3.3.1 Healthcare Requirements

The implementation of an mHealth system is driven by the needs to cut healthcare costs and promote "personal health systems" in the sense of higher levels of healthcare personalization and a more active role of patients in their health management [2]. For mHealth ECG monitoring, this can be achieved by ECG body sensors. With such sensors, a part of the monitoring outcomes can be made available to the patients themselves. Furthermore, patients can be given some control over the devices used in the measurement. In other words, an appropriate user interface can make the difference between a product used only by enthusiasts or a niche of professionals, and a product intended for the general population.

Next, making the user interface user-friendly should be one of the primary goals. For example, seniors are more likely to develop critical health conditions and would benefit the most from the availability of healthcare services at home. Seniors are in general less tech-savvy than the average population and therefore feel less comfortable when using modern technology, which they usually consider unintuitive. As a result, as a recent study says, "Digital health is not reaching most seniors" [3]. Therefore, an mHealth system should be designed with seniors in mind—to be simple and intuitive also for them, and to be able to provide only relevant information or alerts to specific users.

User friendliness should be the key goal in software development, since it could be crucial for the acceptance of the mHealth solutions. Another software development goal should be easy integration of the system into users' everyday lives, which can further increase user acceptance. The system should thus be smart, i.e., interconnected into the network of existing devices and into the everyday routines of its users. Various social networks and the existing ecosystems of healthcare devices, applications and behaviors should also be considered. Finally, the option of future expansions should be left open.

The smartphone application has already been identified as an important part of the mHealth system, because it represents a user interface to the entire system. Nowadays, it can be considered also a very convenient one, since smartphones are becoming an increasingly large part of users' lives, and because they can provide interconnection with other services and applications, and means for automated upgrades and expansions. Since the mobile application is such an important part of the mHealth system and offers so many opportunities, it is described in more detail in the following subsection.

3.3.2 Smartphone Application

We begin this section by describing the basic functionalities of the smartphone in an mHealth system: data storage and visualization, data transmission to other parts of the mHealth system, and user alerting. The description will be general and should

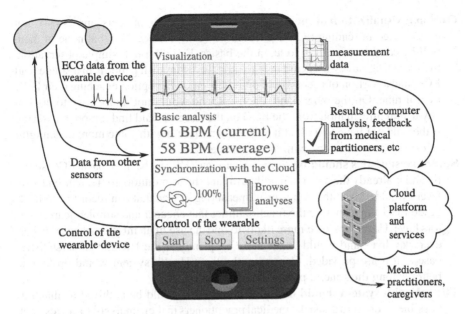

Fig. 3.2 Schematic presentation of the basic smartphone functionality in an mHealth system for ECG monitoring

hold for all mHealth application. Next, we shall focus on ECG monitoring. Figure 3.2 gives a schematic presentation of the basic smartphone functionality in an mHealth system for ECG monitoring.

According to the mHealth requirements, the measured data on the smartphone should be available to the patients themselves as well as to the medical practitioners. A good way of sharing the data among involved parties is having the smartphone process and display the data to the user in real time and in a user-friendly fashion, while also forwarding the unprocessed data to the Cloud via an Internet connection. How the data should be transferred to the Cloud is not well defined and there are not many requirements regarding that functionality. The data could be sent either in near real-time (with minimal delay) or in larger packets, for example once per hour, once per day, etc. Data transmission could be fully automatic or under patient's control. The transmitted data could contain only manually approved segments of measurement or all the gathered data. The data could also be processed prior to transmission to the Cloud, to lower the data transmission and to limit the transfer only to relevant statistics. It all largely depends on the purpose of the monitoring.

Some reasonable requirements for the mHealth mobile application for ECG monitoring, also given in Fig. 3.2, are:

A familiar user interface. The software on the smartphone can use an interface design that is familiar to the user, and will thus require very little effort from the user to master it.

Optional visualization of the measurements. Although patients are usually not experienced in reading ECGs, it would be wrong to speculate that none of them will be capable or willing to learn the basics. Even through simple observation, the more tech-savvy users are able to quickly distinguish patterns in a single lead ECG and a portion of users would definitely enjoy the option of seeing their ECG in real time. On the other hand, the users who would not find it easy to discern any useful information from the ECG on the screen would find it more reassuring if they did not have to look at it and could replace it with some more meaningful information, for starters, with the heart rate value.

Standard statistics should be shown. Heart rate (HR) is the most basic ECG statistic and is already the norm in readily available heart monitors for recreational use. Users would expect that a powerful measuring device that can record a medical-grade ECG can also have the functionalities that cheaper and simpler heart monitors have. Users would be more likely to find the use of an mHealth device in their everyday lives and would use it more frequently if the HR and some statistics based on it are provided. Consequently, the mHealth system would proliferate better among the general public.

The mHealth system should use the Cloud. Data should be archived as much as possible, in order to assist the medical practitioners in their analysis, to aid research and to enable the extraction of new knowledge from the long-term measurements, Cloud services seem perfect for data storage, since they also facilitate the sharing of data. The archived data will become also an indispensable source of information, once the fully automatic analyses reach maturity. Having the data readily available on the Cloud will shorten the research time and enable faster integration of newly developed algorithms and procedures into operational use.

The ambient data should be analyzed. The ECG measurements have limited value if no additional information on the patient and its activity is available; e.g., the absolute value of the HR is only slightly informative, unless the patient's age and the current physical activity are also known. Furthermore, when alerting is provided, the ambient data should be included in the real-time analysis before any kind of alerting takes place. For example, an alert "Your beat rate has been 150 BPM for 30 min, this could be a dangerous situation!" could be made much smarter if an activity information is also provided: "You have been running for half an hour, your beat rate is steady at 150 BPM, keep up the good work!"

The ECG body sensor should be fully controlled by the smartphone. The general population is already familiar with the smartphone user interface and using it would make the mHealth users more comfortable with the ECG body sensor. At the same time, it would greatly simplify the ECG body sensor itself, as it would relax its requirements for human inputs and outputs, such as buttons, switches, LEDs and displays.

A configurable alerting system should be provided. If life-threatening conditions are detected, the application should alert either the user, a nearby healthcare provider, or lastly the emergency department. The software could also provide an assistance in a situation of medical emergency, to any of the pre-mentioned actors in the mHealth system. In the simplest case, the assistance could be in the form of instructions on how to handle the patient in the detected situation, while a more sophisticated application could measure the patient's vital signals and display them on the smartphone screen to aid the actors on the scene. Nevertheless, each case would have to be tailored to the specific area of use and the specifics of the mHealth device in question.

There are many other requirements and implementation details, related to the interface design, the ability of tailoring for different technical skills, the local estimation and graphic representation of the measured parameters, etc., that would differentiate the future mHealth applications.

3.4 An Example of an ECG Monitoring System

In this section, a tentative design of an mHealth system for long-term ECG monitoring of patients or healthy and health-proactive individuals is presented. Several options for the implementation of such a system using state-of-the-art technology are considered. We pay attention to the fulfillment of the mHealth requirements and making the system appealing both to its users and to medical practitioners. Finally, we envision that such a system will have broader benefits and will ultimately help to advance the science.

The design of the system takes into account the existing technical standards, allowing easy connection of various ECG body sensors and their immediate replacement if an improved version becomes available. Besides the ECG sensor, the system architecture allows inclusion of additional sensors, on the same device or on additional devices, if such additions prove useful for monitoring the patient's condition in the future. For example, sensors for remote monitoring of respiratory acoustic phenomena (cough, obstruction) or sensors for activity detection would complement the ECG sensor nicely.

The immediate use of the mHealth system can be based on the visual observation of selected critical vital parameters and their recent changes. Through such observation, it is possible to evaluate the effectiveness of a treatment and to foresee a possible deterioration in advance. In the future, after a thorough research of the area, automatic analysis will be able to complement or even replace the visual inspection of the vital parameters. We foresee that alarms will be implemented to alert the medical practitioners on the high possibility of deterioration before the monitored parameter will reach a critical value. Based on the simultaneous evaluation of multiple variables, the automatic analysis will provide the threat level and its trend in the form of the modified early warning score (MEWS) [4]. The analysis of the vital functions in a longer time period will allow for the implementation of cognitive methods; for example, fully personalized analysis of a cardiogram over a longer time period will be used as an input for determining the patient's threat level [5].

As described previously, the device that would act as a crucial link between the mHealth system components should be carried around by the user, should have computing and communication capabilities, and should be unobtrusive to the user. Today, such a device already exists, namely the smartphone. Smartphones are already owned by more than 2 billion people and their number is still growing. The smartphone connects to the ECG body sensor via the low-power wireless Bluetooth Smart protocol [6] and records everything that the ECG body sensor measures. Besides being extremely low-power, this protocol offers sufficient bandwidth for ECG data streams, concurrent communication with multiple sensors and data encryption.

For security, the measured data stored on the personal smartphone does not contain any information that could facilitate identification of the user. The transfer of the data to the Cloud is encrypted and largely depersonalized—no personal data other than the measurement is ever transmitted to the Cloud. No other personal data is actually required to be stored on the Cloud; aside from the users themselves, only authorized medical practitioners possess additional personal information of the user, such as the health record. The access to the data stored in the Cloud is handled through accounts of varying permissions, which are managed with a safe and reliable account management system. Customized interfaces can be provided for various medical practitioner profiles, to aid them in using, viewing and analyzing the data. These interfaces are managed by the same account management system as the data permissions. Private users also get access to a custom interface for accessing their own data, although they may prefer to use only their personal terminal, without ever connecting to the Cloud.

Another important part of mHealth systems will be open interfaces for custom-made applications and add-ons that communicate either with the Cloud or the smartphone. Such add-ons might end up with discovering a more suitable representation of the measured data for the laymen, or increasing the options for the patients to monitor their vital functions. The options for using the measured data are endless, but interfaces for accessing it will have to be approached with due caution, since sensitive personal data are at stake and should be protected with great care. For example, it may be feasible to identify individuals based on an advanced analysis of the data from the ECG sensor in the near future. When designing an mHealth system, such options can be seen as both drawback and opportunity.

3.5 Smartphone Application Challenges

The ubiquitous smartphones (also tablets, soon-to-follow smart watches, and other smart wearables) have well defined interfaces to which a large portion of the general population is already familiar with. To be acceptable to users, the mHealth mobile application should follow the guidelines set by existing and widely accepted smartphone applications; i.e., the guidelines set by the behavior of various popular software applications, their integration with the smartphone hardware and other software, and their ways of interfacing with the user. Therefore, to integrate better with the user's everyday activities, the following guidelines are recognized for the smartphone application used in an mHealth system, based on the feedback from volunteering users of an early mHealth prototype system:

Ease of use. The users' expectations for the applications on their smartphones are increasingly strict. Applications must be installed in a standard and simple manner, set-up in a few clicks (if at all), and then executed as the user would expect. That is, if the user expects the application to start ECG measurement, then the application should do just that, without requiring the user to go through a lot of menus, settings or input boxes.

The ability to run in the background. That is, the ability to perform measurements, analyze them in real time for the requirements of the user interface, and transfer them to the Cloud to be stored, all while the smartphone screen is off.

Low-power requirements. The mobile application must respect the limitations of the battery-powered smartphone, and must not significantly increase the need for the smartphone to be charged.

Integration of the alerting system. The smartphone's operating system implements a built-in messaging, notification and alerting sub-system, which is familiar to the users and allows for the alerts to be presented in a user-defined manner.

Adjustable level of user engagement. The mobile application should target a wide range of people and their willingness to engage their time into the ECG measurement. Besides using the adjustable notifications system familiar to the user, the application should be able to adjust to the user's wishes in other areas too. Examples of adjustable features are: the level of the displayed details and the frequency of the relevant information updates, or the way the synchronization with the Cloud works (always, or only over WiFi, or only when charging, etc.).

A keen observer might notice that the last guideline seems to contradict the first one. It does not need to, though, since applications can be made very adaptable to their users. Therefore, to adhere to both guidelines, the default application behavior is first tuned to the needs of a basic user with a limited desire for engagement with the system. Then, through the provided settings, the application can be configured to show more data and allow more details to be fine-tuned. Thus, the application is made simple for the basic users, while allowing the more advanced users, who are willing to fiddle with the settings, to enable more control for themselves.

Although a proper user interface design would take care of most of the mentioned guidelines, some aspects remain to be tackled with the back-end logic. When designing their own ECG monitoring system, the authors of this book have been presented with four main challenges:

- transmission of the measured data from the ECG body sensor to a smartphone,
- synchronization of time clocks between the ECG body sensor and the smartphone,
- storage of measurements, and
- detection of heartbeats and heart rate calculation.

All of them are discussed in the following subsections.

3.5.1 Transmission of Measured Data to the Smartphone

The most basic functionality of the mHealth-enabled ECG body sensor is the ability to record ECG measurements. The design goals of the ECG body sensor dictate low weight and extremely low power consumption, and thus constrain the ECG body sensor capabilities. One of the several trade-offs that can be made in the ECG body sensor design is the approach for storing the measurements. Measurements can be either stored on-board, as done in [7], or they can be transferred in real time to another device, such as the user's smartphone, as done in [8].

While the use of on-board storage should be (if properly implemented) simpler, more energy efficient, more error tolerant, and completely self-reliant, it is hard to consolidate it with the requirements of an mHealth system. To empower the patient, the measurements should be accessible to the patient in near real-time. In contrast, transferring the measurement to the smartphone in real time, e.g., over a radio connection, enables real-time access to the measurements and thus easier integration into the mHealth system. The price for it, however, are higher power consumption, a more complex overall system, the need to synchronize the ECG body sensor and the smartphone, and the reliance of the ECG body sensor on the external hardware, e.g., the smartphone or some other data gateway.

The radio transfer can also be arbitrarily complex. In the simplest form, it would consist only of data sampling followed by broadcasting the samples through a radio transmitter. A more elaborated form could comprise complex data sampling, data caching on-board, transmission of compressed data packets with error correction mechanisms, acknowledgment of all the received packets by the receiver, and retransmission of lost data packets. A hybrid approach that would reap benefits while avoiding the drawbacks of the on-board storage could also be used. This would increase the system complexity, but any additional complexity in the system design that eases the system use should be viewed as perfectly acceptable.

3.5.2 Synchronization of Clocks

The moment the data leaves the measuring device and enters another, the problem of clock synchronization arises. Here we explain why multiple clocks in the system make an issue, and discuss possible ways of alleviating it.

Time keeping is an old problem [9] that has been largely forgotten by the general population in the last decades. The age of Internet has brought the endless manual clock synchronization to a close end, by providing several very accurate clocks which are accessible via the Internet (or via GPS) and enabling automatic software synchronization of our computers with these precise clocks. The above sentence already discloses the gist of the problem—clock synchronization did not go away, it merely became automated on a large portion of machines that we interface with. The smartphone falls under the category of Internet-connected devices. For the time being, we shall, therefore, assume that it does not require any additional clock synchronization. For devices that are not connected to the Internet or other large interconnection networks with centralized time keeping, the clock synchronization remains an issue that needs addressing. The ECG body sensor certainly represents an example of such a device.

The electronic circuits most often use inexpensive quartz crystal oscillators to keep time to a limited precision. The modern quartz oscillators are accurate to under 100 ppm [10], which translates into time keeping devices (clocks) with similar accuracy. A clock that is stable to 100 ppm is also said to be accurate to $24 * 60 * 60/10^{-4} = 8.64$ s per day. Under relatively steady temperature conditions, these oscillators can perform at least an order of magnitude better, that is, they drift for less than 1 s per day. One second is in the same order of magnitude as the length of a single heartbeat, so quartz-based clocks could be considered precise enough for performing short measurements without external clock synchronization. Even for measurements of several days, such error could be considered acceptable if no synchronization with other sensors and devices is required. However, as we describe in the Chap. 2, several concurrent ECG measurements can be merged into even more descriptive forms of ECG, which requires synchronization precise to a hundredth of a second.

ECG body sensors are also miniaturized for a lower weight, and as such usually do not include a real-time clock circuitry with a dedicated battery for time keeping when the device is turned off. They should be reminded of the current time on every start-up or reset. Therefore, two arguments are in favor of synchronizing the ECG body sensor's clock with the smartphone: the need to perform long measurements (on the timescale of several days) and the need to adjust the clock after start-up or reset. Since the ECG body sensor and the smartphone constitute a simple distributed system, the solution is to use one of the many clock synchronization techniques for distributed systems [11]. In such a distributed system, the smartphone has a more accurate time keeping. Therefore, one solution would be to consider its time as a reference, and have the ECG body sensor synchronized to it at all times. This solution, however, may still cause measurements performed on different smartphones to drift in time, and is only appropriate if such drift is acceptable.

3.5.3 Storage of Measurements

One of the essential mHealth functionalities is the storage of measurements, which can be regarded as a two-level process. The first level is implemented on the smartphone, where the measurements are stored until they are uploaded to the Cloud. The second level is on the Cloud, where the measurements are stored as a part of the patients' medical record, knowledge databases, analytical Cloud services and similar. We shall not discuss much about the Cloud part of storage here, since it largely depends on the goals of the particular mHealth system. We shall rather focus on the storage of the measurements while they are stored on the user's smartphone, which makes them easily accessible to the user.

There is a plethora of file formats for storing ECG to choose from, and one should choose very wisely. The file storage should be implemented in a way that adheres to the existing ISO standards of the 22077 family [12–15], related to the storage of ECG measurements. In addition to standards, there are also some mHealth-specific requirements for the storage of measurements, which are in line with the general idea of mHealth—to help make patients more proactive and improve the integration between medical services:

- *The use of files for storing individual measurements and the use of standard file formats whenever possible.*
- *Empowerment of patients*, which can be accomplished by giving users the ability to browse, copy, export and view the measurements with standard tools available. Open file formats present a more rational choice compared to proprietary formats, since the latter would severely limit the users in their access to the measurements, and could cause vendor lock-ins and additional expenses for the developers of mHealth system extensions. A recent review of open file formats has been done in [16], and while a lot of them have been designed with very different ECG measurements in mind, there are several that fulfill quite a lot of the listed requirements.
- *The ability to store various meta data in the same file.* Since the mHealth is in its infancy, it is unreasonable to expect that the meta data structure adopted at the design stage will pass the test of time and the increasing usage. Therefore, the meta data should be at most weakly structured, to allow for future additions or modifications.
- *The ability to store measurement data other than ECG in the same file.* As explained before, the additional measurements will in time be able to provide indispensable information complementary to the ECG, allowing for a far more in-depth analysis and a more precise diagnosis. Like in the case of meta data, trying to identify all data types in advance would not be very prudent. Therefore, a flexible file format supporting additional measurements of varying sample sizes and sampling frequencies would be most welcome.
- *The use of compact file formats* to allow the storage of large data quantities on a standard-size smartphone storage.
- *Robustness of the storage procedures against abrupt and unanticipated interruptions.* The inclusion of personal smartphones into the mHealth hardware scheme is followed by a specific set of problems, which are not inherent to medical devices. The smartphones and the software running on them are not designed for the same degree of reliability as are certified medical devices. Furthermore, they are under full control of their users, who may want to abruptly pause, stop or interfere with the ongoing measurement. While performing measurements, users may also use other applications with a wide range of system resource requirements, which may inadvertently affect these measurements. Therefore, the interruptions in measurements, including those that occur while the mHealth application is in the middle of a file-storing procedure, should be considered normal operation. Either the chosen file formats should be robust enough to allow not-fully written files to remain readable up to the point of corruption, or some other form of file repair

should be available. The latter is less optimal, since it requires a more complex file management system and adds new points of possible system failure.

However, an existing file format that would fully satisfy the listed requirements is impossible to find. Since the novel mHealth systems are coming with their own special requirements, modifying the existing file formats or even designing new ones is a viable option. Here one should not forget the lesson learned from the existence of a plethora of file formats for storing ECG: the design should not be too specific and should allow for future changes and improvements.

3.5.4   Detection of Heartbeats

After a measurement is recorded and the time of individual samples well determined, the processing of the ECG can start. The most basic processing of an ECG signal, intended to derive some information of user interest, is the detection of heartbeats. More precisely, it is the detection of the times when heartbeats occur. The application can then use those times to calculate some basic heartbeat statistics, such as the heart rate [17], or perform more complex processing, such as automatic classification of beats [18]. The heartbeat information is even more useful if it can be accessed in real time. The mobile application can use such data to advise or alert the user when certain conditions are detected. In the cases when the detected conditions appear to be alarming, the mobile application could be used to automatically alert the patient's caregivers or even the nearby emergency department. From an empowered patient's perspective, the heartbeat detection can be used by the patient directly for an easier observation of the heart rhythm and the shape of characteristic ECG waves. For example, proactive patients might be curious about how their heart reacts to changes in their activity, their nutrition or emotional state. They might even learn to better recognize their current condition after they inspect the current heartbeat rhythm and shape.

Although the beat detection is a mature field in science, with plenty of known algorithms to choose from [19], one should note that these algorithms were designed for a different kind of ECG measurements. They were mostly designed to be used on 12-lead ECG measurements made in a controlled environment. As discussed in Chap. 2, the ECG body sensor delivers differential ECGs that differ from the standard conventional ECGs in several details. Furthermore, the ECG body sensor records far more noise than the standard 12-lead ECG apparatus. The additional noise is produced because of the limited number of electrodes, the limited distance between the electrodes, and most importantly, the difficult measurement conditions under which the mHealth system is used. To reach full integration into patients' lives, mHealth devices are being used during everyday activities, in totally uncontrolled environments. When patients are engaged in physical activities and exercise, the amount of noise caused by the muscle activity and the physical strain on the electrode contacts is very high. Moreover, the conditions vary during the measurement. The users are very likely to be partly at rest and partly active during the same measurement. They are also moving in environments with variable electromagnetic interference, ranging from practically zero (e.g. in nature, far from any human-made infrastructure) up to the limits posed by the health standards. All in all, the difficult conditions should be countered by making the algorithms more robust, lowering expectations on the result accuracy, and additional statistics returned by the algorithms, e.g., noise levels.

Several modifications to the known beat detection algorithms should be implemented to make them appropriate for body sensor ECGs:

• Aggressive input filtering aimed at removing all the noise in the measurement. The input filtering can be performed as digital processing for the task of beat detection only.
• Build-in adaptivity to the input signal orientation and to gradual changes in the ECG shape because of baseline wandering, i.e., on a timescale of more than one beat. For example, user's posture will influence the ECG shape, while the varying water content in the skin will influence its electrical conductance and consequently change the amplitude of the ECG. Users might also modify the position of the ECG body sensor during the measurement, and thus change the measured ECG shape completely.
• A measure of signal noise, which can be first used as a help in beat detection, and second, as an additional output information from the beat detector.
• If the ECG body sensor provides also other measurements, e.g. activity or EMG, they can be used as additional information for beat detection.

An important question to think about is also where the beat detection takes place. It should take place close to the user to make the results available for further processing in near real time. It is worth noting though that several seconds of measurement may need to pass before beats can be detected with sufficient probability.

Beat detection could theoretically be done on the Cloud if the measurement is being transferred to the Cloud in real-time. However, this option comes with a severe drawback. When the Cloud is not available, the beat detection will not occur. Therefore, the reliance on the Cloud, which is equivalent to the reliance on a sufficiently fast Internet connection, is unacceptable for the general mHealth application. It might be acceptable for some special cases though, e.g., when monitoring is implemented only within a single health institution.

A better alternative is to perform beat detection on the smartphone or on the ECG body sensor. The smartphone is a device with increasingly large amount of computational power at its disposal, with near real-time access to all the measurement data required by the beat detection algorithm, and thus seems very fitting. The disadvantage of implementing the beat detection on the ECG body sensor, as opposed to the smartphone, are the limited computational capabilities of the ECG body sensor. Furthermore, running a computationally demanding algorithm on the ECG body sensor could seriously increase the power consumption and thus decrease the device autonomy and limit its use. The benefit of detecting the beats on the body sensor, on the other hand, is in the possibility to lower the amount of the data to be sent to the smartphone. Adaptive data compression algorithms may be used before the data is transmitted if beat locations are known; the ECG can be compressed with varying compression ratios for different parts of the ECG signal. The noise level may also be assessed better if beat locations are given, which again enables more control over adaptive compression algorithms. Compressing the data to be sent is very welcome and can be viewed from two different angles. First, it can be seen as a means of lowering the power consumption of the ECG body sensor, since transmitting compressed data usually requires less energy. Second, it can be viewed as an opportunity for the ECG body sensor to gather and transmit more information to the smartphone, since more of the available bandwidth remains accessible. Therefore, selecting the device where the beat detection will be implemented requires deciding on a trade-off between benefits and disadvantages, and may also include hybrid solutions. Nevertheless, getting the most out of the system will require at least some rudimentary beat detection to be implemented on the ECG body sensor itself.

Furthermore, the beat detection can be partly done on the smartphone or body sensor and partly extended to the Cloud, where all the patient's measurement history and healthcare information is stored. Such a hybrid solution would make the most precise beat detection available to medical practitioners through the Cloud services, while also making the preliminary beat detection available to the user of the mHealth system. Extending the hybrid solution from beat detection to complete ECG processing would be a natural next step. At this point, one could even make a case for distributed computing, where the processing workload of the Cloud service for ECG processing is lowered on the account of the users' smartphones performing the bulk of the processing in advance. This, however, is a topic for further research and experimentation.

3.6 Example Algorithms

In this section, the complex task of heart rate calculation is examined and an algorithm for heart rate calculation is proposed. A schematic representation of the proposed HR calculation algorithm is shown in Fig. 3.3. Starting with a raw ECG input (step 1), the first part is the beat detection composed of filtering, extraction of extrema, estimation of spike likelihood and peak detection (steps 2 to 5). Then follows the noise estimation—the noise in the vicinity of detected beats is estimated and beats from noisy parts of the signal are discarded from further processing (step 6). Lastly, beat-to-beat intervals are measured (step 7), outliers removed, and the remaining intervals averaged to derive HR (step 8).

The first task—beat detection—is based on an algorithm [17] designed for use in an mHealth system. The proposed beat detection algorithm is in many aspects similar to previously known algorithms [19], but designed to work on differential ECGs with a low sample rate and a low signal-to-noise ratio. Furthermore, it is not affected by the orientation of the ECG features, since it searches only for rapid changes in the input signal, ignoring their exact nature. It was designed to have a small memory footprint

Fig. 3.3 A schematic representation of the HR calculation algorithm

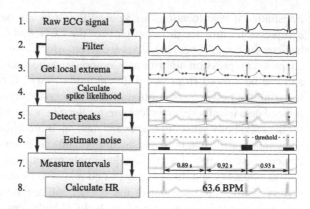

1. Raw ECG signal
2. Filter
3. Get local extrema
4. Calculate spike likelihood
5. Detect peaks
6. Estimate noise — — — — — — — — threshold — — —
7. Measure intervals | 0.89 s | 0.92 s | 0.93 s |
8. Calculate HR   63.6 BPM

and to use as little processing power as possible, so that it could be implemented on the ECG body sensor.

3.6.1 Filtering

The beat detection algorithm is tuned to detect only the QRS complex, because it is the most prominent feature of almost any ECG and is far less sensitive to morphological changes than the other ECG waves [20]. The frequency spectrum of the QRS is quite limited. A narrow frequency band filter that would pass only the QRS frequencies, e.g. 10–40 Hz [21], could be used to remove all noise in the frequency bands which carry no ECG-related information. Filtering is performed using a digital filter only in the beat detection phase. The filtered signal is later discarded. Therefore, the filter used in this step does not deform the measurement and is used only to help the beat detection task. For simpler and more efficient implementation, a low-pass filter is used with the threshold set at 45 Hz. The filter is implemented as Brown's exponential smoothing [22], also called exponential moving average (EMA).

Brown's exponential smoothing calculates the smoothed value $s(t_n)$ of a sampled signal $x(t_n)$ for each time step t_n as:

$$s(t_0) = x(t_0)$$
$$\Delta t = t_{n-1} - t_n$$
$$\alpha = 1 - e^{\frac{\Delta t}{\tau}}$$
$$s(t_n) = \alpha x(t_n) + (1 - \alpha)s(t_{n-1}), \qquad (3.1)$$

where α is a smoothing factor, derived from the time constant τ that specifies the time in which the smoothed response to a unit step input would reach the value $1 - 1/e$. Δt is the time step, which does not need to be constant throughout the measurement.

3.6.2 Extrema Extraction

The local extrema of the filtered ECG signal are extracted to lower the amount of the data that has to be processed in the following steps and thus simplify further processing. Local extrema, i.e. positive and negative peaks, are the positions in which the derivative changes its sign. They appear in an alternate fashion, with each minimum followed by a maximum, and vice-versa.

From the interval of a monotonic input signal between each pair of consecutive extrema, a single extremum in the derivative is also extracted. Based on the derivative sign, the extracted extremum is either a minimum (negative sign) or a maximum (positive sign). For example, from the interval between a minimum peak and a maximum peak in the input signal, the input signal is non-decreasing, the derivative is non-negative and, therefore, a maximum in the derivative is extracted.

3.6.3 Spike Likelihood Estimation

The term spike will be used here to refer to a rapid change in the signal amplitude— either up or down, followed by a rapid change in the other direction. For more distinct changes in amplitude, the spike will be termed as strong. The QRS complex contains at least one strong spike, regardless of where the ECG is measured and thus independent of the ECG body sensor placement and orientation. Therefore the beat detection can be implemented by spike detection.

A spike contains a local extremum as its peak. In this algorithm step, each local extremum is tested to determine if it represents the peak of a strong spike. Spike likelihood is introduced as a measure of spike strength in each local extremum. The estimation takes three signal extrema and two signal derivative extrema as input, and converts them into a unit-less number. For each signal extremum, the likelihood is calculated as:

$$a \cdot b \cdot c \cdot d,$$

where a is the difference in amplitudes of the given and the previous extremum, b is the difference in amplitudes of the given and the next extremum, and c and d are the derivative extrema to the left and to the right of the given extremum. A graphical explanation of the likelihood estimation step is given in Fig. 3.4.

A part of an ECG input signal with a strong spike is shown in Fig. 3.4 with a solid line. For every triplet of extrema in the input signal, extracted in the previous algorithm step and marked with small circles, two pairs of parameters are calculated. The first two parameters, a and b, marked with double-ended arrows, are obtained as amplitude differences between two consecutive input signal extrema as follows: a is the difference in amplitudes between the second and the first extremum, b is the difference in amplitudes between the third and the second extremum. The other two parameters, c and d, marked with single-ended arrows, are obtained as extrema of

Fig. 3.4 Likelihood
estimation scheme on an
example of a strong spike

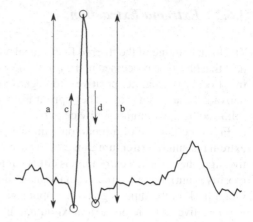

corresponding positive and negative signal derivatives: c is the maximum derivative of the input signal between the first and the second extremum of the input signal, d is the minimum derivative of the input signal between the second and the third extremum of the input signal.

3.6.4 Peak Detection

High likelihood values are assumed to be caused by strong spikes in the input signal, which in turn are a sign of significant probability for a QRS complex in the signal. Therefore, the spike likelihood could be taken by its absolute value; an absolute threshold, with values high enough, could be applied as a filter. Nevertheless, to achieve some adaptability, spike likelihood is rather observed relative to its previous peak values.

First, modified exponential smoothing is applied on the likelihood and the result is multiplied with a constant factor f. The result is called dynamic threshold $d(t_n)$. The best values for f are in the interval from 1 to 10, which was confirmed by a preliminary analysis on different ECG input signals. Second, as the input signal is processed in real time, the local peaks of likelihood are compared with the dynamic threshold value. When a likelihood value higher than the dynamic threshold is encountered, a peak is detected and the following two procedures take place: the threshold value is set to the value of the likelihood in the new peak and the detected heartbeat is the output from the algorithm. Formally, the peak detection algorithm can be written as follows:

$$d(t_n) = f \cdot s(t_{n-1})$$

$$s(t_n) = \begin{cases} \text{as calculated in Eq. 3.1,} & \text{if } \left(x(t_n) \leq d(t_n)\right) \\ x(t_n), & \text{otherwise.} \end{cases} \qquad (3.2)$$

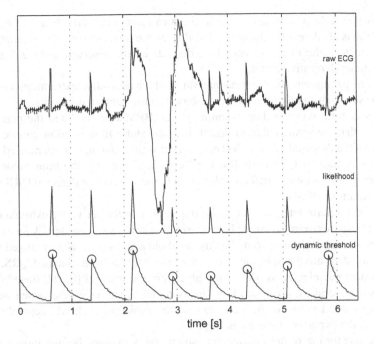

Fig. 3.5 ECG signal from a significantly distorted body surface measurement (*top*), spike likelihood estimated for the ECG signal (*middle*), dynamic threshold (*bottom*). The circles on the bottom plot mark the detected beats. The Y axis is not marked, since its absolute values are not relevant

The described peak detection algorithm step is fully adaptable to the input signal and detects only the highest peaks on a time scale that is controlled by the parameter τ. An output of this step is also the result of the complete beat detection algorithm, which is represented by the timing of QRS complexes in the input ECG signal.

Figure 3.5 shows an example of the likelihood estimation and dynamic thresholding on a segment of a significantly distorted ECG signal. In the figure, it can be seen that the peaks in spike likelihood correspond to the locations of QRS complexes in the ECG signal. The QRS complex of the fourth beat is properly detected, even though it is significantly distorted by noise. The performance of the described beat detection algorithm is further confirmed by correct exclusion of the spike-shaped noise between the fifth and the sixth beat of the ECG measurement.

3.6.5 *Noise Estimator*

In this section, we describe a crude noise estimator. The estimation is done by counting the number of large first derivative extrema in the area close to a detected beat. These are likely to be caused by noise and could disturb the beat detector. This estimator is thus able to estimate noise in the area around detected beats, in order to discard the beats detected with low reliability on the noisy signal. The estimator has two parameters: the time interval where derivatives are observed and the threshold amplitude for derivative extrema.

The first parameter, i.e., the time interval in which derivative extrema are counted, could be set dynamically for each beat—based on the heart rate, or statically—using a fixed size time window. For example, if 200 BPM is considered the maximum heart rate that the system should detect, then the static time window can be set to the time of the detected QRS ± 300 ms, since this time window is guaranteed not to overlap with another QRS complex. For the dynamic setting, the time window not overlapping with another QRS complex is set to the time of the detected QRS ± 500 ms * (60/current BPM).

The second parameter, i.e., the threshold amplitude for derivative extrema (β), is used to classify extrema as either large or small, where only large are likely to cause problems in beat detection. To make this threshold adaptable, β is normalized by the largest first derivative amplitude within the time interval of the located QRS. Thus the β should be selected as a relative value from the interval [0...1]. Based on the analysis of several experimental ECG measurements, we have determined that 0.5 is usually a good value for β. Nevertheless, the choice of β should depend on the amount of the expected noise in the signal.

Some fine tuning of both parameters should be performed before implementing the algorithm on a specific ECG body sensor and for a specific range of expected ECG input signals.

3.6.6   Heart Rate Calculation

The frequency of heartbeats—the heart rate (HR)—is calculated on a short time interval and reported as the number of beats per minute (BPM). Although it sounds straightforward, robust calculation of heart rate is difficult when the measurement is noisy. The presented real-time algorithm for HR calculation works by averaging the intervals between successive beats. It is thus able to return a new heart rate value for each newly detected beat.

A list of beats is maintained while the measurement is in progress, with the following procedures applied to each detected beat:

1. The output of the noise estimator is taken to discard beats that were detected while noise levels were above the threshold. If the estimated noise is above 5, i.e., five spikes of comparative amplitude were identified near the QRS, then this beat time is discarded due to high noise and the procedure ends here. Otherwise, the beat time is added to the list of beats.
2. The list of beats is trimmed to contain only the beats from the last S seconds of the measurement, by checking the age of each beat in the list and removing those of an age more than S. The time window S is a parameter that should be adjusted

to suit the system requirements. Since the unit of HR is in beats per minute, an appropriate value for S is 60 (1 min). Lower values will make the calculation more sensitive to changes in the HR, but also more susceptible to noise.

To enable reliable results when noisy data is used, only the most reliable beat-to-beat intervals are used for averaging. For example, if a beat is not detected due to noise (false negative), this creates a longer-than-average beat-to-beat interval. Similarly, if the noise in the signal is falsely recognized as a beat (false positive), this creates two shorter-than-average beat-to-beat intervals. Such intervals should be detected and handled properly to eliminate their influence on the mean HR. The full procedure for processing the list of beats is as follows:

1. The differences between all consecutive beats in the list are calculated, to obtain a list of beat-to-beat intervals.
2. The mean beat-to-beat interval is calculated from the beat-to-beat interval list.
3. Those beat-to-beat interval outliers which deviate from the mean by more than D are removed from the list. The value of D should be 50% or higher, otherwise false positives might not be detected.
4. If less than N beat-to-beat intervals remain, the procedure is exited with an error indication. This check enforces that at least N intervals are averaged for a more accurate and more stable estimate. Higher values of N will result in a smoother evolution of HR through time and should be preferred. Formally, N is down-limited by 1 (at least one beat-to-beat interval is required to calculate the heart rate) and up-limited by the minimal number of beats that can be detected in S seconds. The upper limit is thus a function of the minimal heart rate and largely depends on the intended use of the system.
5. The value of HR is calculated as (60/mean beat-to-beat interval).
6. The resulting HR value is then checked against the physical bounds for the human HR. Very broad limits for HR, e.g. [20–250], can be selected, so that this last check filters only the extreme periodic noise, such as the electric mains noise that can appear on disconnected electrodes of the ECG body sensor.

If no error occurs, the calculated HR can be shown to the user (preferably rounded to the nearest integer) or used for further analysis. Otherwise, an indication that the HR cannot be reliably detected should be shown to the user.

The HR display should furthermore reflect the cases when no heartbeats have been detected in some time (e.g., in 10 s). This should not be a cause for alarm, since these cases are not necessarily caused by a cardiac arrest, but far more likely by disconnected electrodes. At this point, the cause for absent beats can be further analyzed, if measurements complementary to the ECG are also available from the sensor. An indicator often used to discern whether the electrodes are attached or not is the measurement of the electrical resistance between the electrodes; infinite resistance implies that the electrodes are not attached, while near-zero resistance implies a short circuit between the electrodes caused, for example, by submerging the sensor in water. Both cases indicate an improper ECG body sensor usage.

Finally, the calculated HR could be written in a file, to complement the ECG measurement. It could, however, be used only for providing an immediate information to the user; after all, a more advanced beat detection and heart rate calculation can be performed off-line, when necessary. The choice whether to store HR information or not is in the designer's hands, because it represents a trade-off between additional storage requirements and the ability to quickly visualize and search through the HR values of past measurements.

References

1. Rashkovska, A., Tomašić, I., Trobec, R.: A telemedicine application: ECG data from wireless body sensors on a smartphone. In: Proceedings of MEET & GVS on the 34th International Convention MIPRO 2011, vol. 1, 2011, pp. 293–296
2. European Commision, Green Paper on mobile health ("mHealth") (2014). https://ec.europa.eu/digital-single-market/en/news/green-paper-mobile-health-mhealth
3. Levine, D.M., Lipsitz, S.R., Linder, J.A.: Trends in seniors' use of digital health technology in the United States, 2011–2014. JAMA **316**(5), 538–540 (2016)
4. Subbe, C., Kruger, M., Rutherford, P., Gemmel, L.: Validation of a modified early warning score in medical admissions. Qjm **94**(10), 521–526 (2001)
5. R. Miller, Rise of the machines: Computers construct better biomarkers (2011). http://www.medscape.com/viewarticle/751079
6. Decuir, J.: Introducing bluetooth smart: Part II: applications and updates. IEEE Consumer Electron. Mag. **3**(2), 25–29 (2014)
7. Saadi, D., Sørensen, H., Hansen, I., Egstrup, K., Jennum, P., Hoppe, K.: ePatch®—A Clinical Overview, Technical report, Technical University of Denmark, Denmark, annual report (2014)
8. Trobec, R., Avbelj, V., Rashkovska, A.: Multi-functionality of wireless body sensors. The IPSI BgD Trans. Internet Res. **10**, 23–27 (2014)
9. Lamport, L.: Time, clocks, and the ordering of events in a distributed system. Commun. ACM **21**(7), 558–565 (1978)
10. Lam, C.S.: A review of the recent development of MEMS and crystal oscillators and their impacts on the frequency control products industry. In: Proceedings of the IEEE International Ultrasonics Symposium, 2008, pp. 694–704
11. Horauer, M.: Clock synchronization in distributed systems, Südwestdeutscher Verlag für Hochschulschriften SVH (2009)
12. Health informatics—medical waveform format—part 1: Encoding rules, Standard ISO/TS 22077-1:2015. International Organization for Standardization, Geneva, Switzerland (2015)
13. Health informatics—medical waveform format—part 3: Electrocardiography, Standard ISO/TS 22077-2:2015, International Organization for Standardization, Geneva, Switzerland (2015)
14. Health informatics—medical waveform format—part 3: Long term electrocardiography, Standard ISO/TS 22077-3:2015, International Organization for Standardization, Geneva, Switzerland (2015)
15. Health informatics—medical waveform format—part 4: Stress test electrocardiography, Standard ISO/TS 22077-4, International Organization for Standardization, Geneva, Switzerland (2015)
16. Trigo, J.D., Alesanco, Á., Martínez, I., García, J.: A review on digital ECG formats and the relationships between them. IEEE Trans. Inf. Technol. Biomed. **16**(3), 432–444 (2012)
17. Lavrič, P., Depolli, M.: Robust beat detection on noisy differential ECG. In: 39th International Convention on Information and Communication Technology, Electronics and Microelectronics, MIPRO 2016, Opatija, Croatia, May 30–June 3, 2016, 2016, pp. 381–386

18. Rashkovska, A., Kocev, D., Trobec, R.: Clustering of heartbeats from ECG recordings obtained with wireless body sensors. In: 39th International Convention on Information and Communication Technology, Electronics and Microelectronics, MIPRO 2016, Opatija, Croatia, May 30–June 3, 2016, 2016, pp. 461–466
19. Kohler, B.-U., Hennig, C., Orglmeister, R.: The principles of software QRS detection. IEEE Eng. Med. Biol. Mag. 21(1), 42–57 (2002)
20. Avbelj, V., Trobec, R., Gersak, B.: Beat-to-beat repolarisation variability in body surface electrocardiograms. Med. Biol. Eng. Comput. 41(5), 556–560 (2003)
21. Buendía-Fuentes, F., Arnau-Vives, M., Arnau-Vives, A., Jiménez-Jiménez, Y., Rueda-Soriano, J., Zorio-Grima, E., Osa-Sáez, A., Martínez-Dolz, L., Almenar-Bonet, L., Palencia-Pérez, M.: High-bandpass filters in electrocardiography: source of error in the interpretation of the ST segment. ISRN Cardiol. (2012)
22. Brown, R.G.: Exponential smoothing for predicting demand. In: Operations Research, vol. 5, pp. 145–145

Chapter 4
ECG Pilot Studies

Abstract The use of wireless ECG body sensors in two pilot studies is presented. The first study, running at the Department of Cardiovascular Surgery of the University Medical Centre Ljubljana, is focused on the investigation of postoperative atrial fibrillation. The patients are monitored with wireless ECG body sensors one day before and five days after the surgery. The second study has been established at the primary care level in the Community Health Centre Ljubljana, with the intention to establish heart rhythm screening. As both studies are still in progress, we present just their setup and some interesting findings that emerged in their starting phase. Based on evidences from long-term ECG measurements, we identify several still open ECG research questions that could utilize the vast amount of long ECG recordings obtained from the pilot studies.

4.1 Motivation

An unobtrusive and lightweight ECG body sensor can be used for long monitoring of the heart's activity in many different situations. The unobtrusiveness is the key for long-term use. In medicine, the term patient means a person under health care, however, at the same time, a patient also means "someone who suffers". With an appropriately designed system, the measuring procedure should not impose additional suffering. The wireless ECG sensor used in the two pilot systems approaches this goal in the sense that "a patient can be less patient".

The long-lasting collaboration between the Jožef Stefan Institute and the University Medical Centre Ljubljana (UMCL) in the research field of electrocardiology has resulted in many publications [1–10]. Among them, several are on the topic of cardiac rhythms before and after cardiac surgery. As postoperative atrial fibrillation (AF) is a common complication after cardiac surgery, the Department of Cardiovascular Surgery at the UMCL decided to conduct a prospective biomedical research study about it. The study was approved by the National Medical Ethics Committee of the Republic of Slovenia in 2015.

On the other hand, there has not been a previous collaboration between the Jožef Stefan Institute and the Community Health Centre Ljubljana (CHCL) in the field

© The Author(s) 2018
R. Trobec et al., *Body Sensors and Electrocardiography*, SpringerBriefs
in Applied Sciences and Technology, DOI 10.1007/978-3-319-59340-1_4

of cardiology. The possibility for collaboration emerged in the last years, when we realized that the use of smartphones (or tablets) can bring the ECG monitoring to everyone who needs it in a simple, safe and affordable way. The initial study [11] started with 13 volunteers for validation of the measurement protocol that was subsequently supplemented. The final goal of the study is to find out if several days of ECG monitoring at home, by using an unobtrusive ECG body sensor, can lead to an earlier evidence-based decision about anamnestic suspicion for cardiac rhythm disturbances.

The research of cardiac electrophysiology could benefit from the vast amount of ECG data that will emerge from broad use of ECG sensors. Some of the interesting research questions on ECG are: what is the real origin of the T wave; what is the origin of the U wave; is there only one sinus node or are there active regions in the atria that perform pacemaking function; what is behind the sick sinus syndrome; can we predict the onset of AF. We tangle some of them in the last section, where we present a few examples from the first steps of the pilot studies.

4.2   Atrial Fibrillation After Cardiac Surgery—A Study at the University Medical Centre Ljubljana

Postoperative AF (POAF) is a complication that often emerges after cardiac surgery. It can result in many health-related complications and in the need for increased healthcare resources. The findings in prediction and prevention of POAF in the last years are not enough to resolve the problem and there is still some uncertainty about the risk stratification and the management of POAF. As reported recently [12], the Department of Cardiovascular Surgery at the UMCL extended a previous study [5, 7] and introduced a new clinical study about the mechanisms of AF, to determine the dynamics of the heart rhythm and the electrophysiological properties of the heart after cardiac operation.

The clinical study utilizes wireless ECG monitoring after surgery for the evaluation of malignancies of the rhythm and the estimation of electrophysiological properties. Within the first stage of the study, a tablet showing the current heart rhythm is posted near the patient's bed and the analysis of the measured ECG is done afterward by a trained expert with computer-supported assistance. If the study is able to demonstrate that online monitoring with automatic recognition of certain events is beneficial, the required functionality will be implemented in the monitoring system to provide online analysis. The wireless ECG monitoring starts one day before surgery and lasts until the fifth postoperative day. AF is expected to occur in some patients in this time frame. It is supposed that such long-term monitoring and analysis of the obtained recordings could enable preventive activity before the start of the expected AF. The activity is planned for implementation in the second stage of the study.

4.2.1 Participation in the Study

The candidates for inclusion in the study are patients anticipated for elective cardiac surgery in the sinus rhythm and patients with expected surgical ablation of AF alone or together with other cardiac surgery. Excluded are: patients with a cardiac pacemaker, urgent cardiac surgery or previous open-heart surgery.

4.2.2 Procedures

One day before surgery, 20 min of high-resolution standard 12-lead ECG recording is obtained for short-term heart rate variability analysis and standard ECG analysis. In the same time, a wireless ECG sensor with two electrodes is placed on the patient's chest for obtaining one-day basal ECG status. The ECG sensor is removed during the surgery and placed again after the surgery for five days. The placement of the sensor is critical, because there is a postoperative wound on the chest and the atrial P wave should be clearly visible. The ECG is recorded on a tablet computer near the patient and also shown on the tablet for the medical practitioners. During the 6-day measurements, an irritation on the skin under the electrodes is possible. In such a case, the ECG sensor should be moved to another position on the body. The tablet is connected to the mains adapter all the time, while the ECG sensor has enough autonomy for the whole period of measurement.

After a 6-day period, the ECG recordings are transferred to a secure computer server for further visual inspection by a medical expert. The goal is to identify the AF burden, e.g. the number and the duration of AF periods. This procedure is described in more detail in the next section. It is expected that such long-term ECG measurements, and other data obtained during the study, will help to better understand the evolution of POAF and the re-emerging of AF after the surgical procedure. With better recordings and understanding of AF, there is a possibility of predicting the risk for AF, which could lead us to use preventive strategies in the identified groups.

4.3 Heart Rhythm Screening—A Study at the Community Health Centre Ljubljana

The pilot study was designed recently at the primary care level at the CHCL, which is taking care for more than 440.000 registered patients. We hope that it will trigger a broad penetration of the ICT into the primary care and also improve the integrated health care with evidence-based decisions. The initial phase of the study [11] tests the pilot protocol within fifteen patients and healthy volunteers. The established study protocol was confirmed in November 2016. Two hundred patients are going to be enrolled, divided randomly in two groups: half of them will wear the ECG body sensor (the test group) and the other half will be maintained according to the classic clinical path (the control group). We expect that the CHCL pilot will provide valuable responses from medical practitioners, patients and caregivers, which can lead to further improvement of the global mHealth system.

4.3.1   Participation in the Study

Patients with no previous diagnosis of heart rhythm disturbances and with an anamnestic suspicion for rhythm disturbance not confirmed previously by a standard 12-lead ECG or Holter ECG are invited to participate in the study. The included patients are further divided in two groups: the test group – where the wireless ECG body sensor is used for 2 days, and the control group – where a standard treatment is taken. The randomized classification of patients into groups is performed by a simple procedure: the first patient is in the test group, the second in the control group, the next one in the test group, and so on. All study participants have to sign an informed written consent before their enrolment.

4.3.2   Procedures

For patients in the test group, the procedure is as follows:

(a) During appointment No. 1, the doctor performs clinical examination and fills in a form with patient's data and anamneses.
(b) The patient receives a diary that he/she will be filling in at home for the period until the next appointment.
(c) The next appointment at the doctor is scheduled after 5–10 days (depending on the capability of the simulation center).
(d) The patient is referred to the simulation center where he/she is equipped with an ECG body sensor, a smartphone and instructions for use.
(e) After two days, the patient returns the ECG sensor and the smartphone to the simulation center—the ECG recording from the smartphone storage is transferred to a secure computer server in the CHCL.
(f) Before appointment No. 2, the doctor examines the patient's ECG recording.
(g) During appointment No. 2, the doctor:

- examines the patient's diary,
- takes appropriate measures: observation, introducing drugs, directing the patient to a clinical specialist, further examinations, or prolongation of the ECG sensor measurement,
- fills the form with results of the clinical examination.

(h) If there was a decision for a prolonged ECG sensor measurement, the doctor proceeds as in (b)–(h). At most two prolongations of the ECG measurement are possible.

For patients in the control group, the procedure is the same as above, except that there are no actions in (d), (e), (f) and (h), because these patients do not use an ECG body sensor.

4.3.3 Simulation Center

A patient comes in the simulation center (SIM) of CHCL to get an ECG body sensor, a smartphone and user instructions. First, the whole procedure is explained by a trained medical technician and then the ECG sensor is placed on the patient's chest at the position where all electrocardiographic waves (P, QRS, T) are clearly visible. There are several standardized sensor positions. The medical technician and the patient find an optimal position, most often with the first attempt, or by testing among a few standardized locations that provide an adequate visibility of the P wave, which is essential for the arrhythmia analysis. The location should be comfortable for the patient and result in an adequate quality of the recorded ECG signal. The patient is instructed how to place the sensor at home, in the case of a bad contact between the electrodes and the skin or in the case of an eventual skin irritation from the electrodes, and where to place the smartphone for a minimally interrupted radio connection. Finally, the patient receives simplified written instructions about all the procedures of the study protocol.

During the initial phase of the study, we have found out that many advanced features of the mobile application, e.g. marking events, inserting comments, generating ECG reports, etc., are not applicable for older patients, who are often not accustomed to use smartphones. Also, several participating volunteers were troubled even by watching the ECG signal—they are not familiar to monitor the ECG during daily activities, when the baseline could be extremely unstable and EMG signals are superimposed to the ECG signal. Based on the patient decision, the SIM center personnel either enables or disables the ECG signal visualization during the measurement. After two days, the patient returns the devices and his diary. The ECG data from the smartphone are transferred to the computer server where an authorized doctor can examine the ECG recording.

4.4 Visual Examination of the ECG Recordings

We have established that the most efficient way to examine a long-term ECG recording is to look over a graphic presentation of the recording in the form of an ECG report (for an example, see Fig. 4.1). Each heartbeat is presented as a thin point with

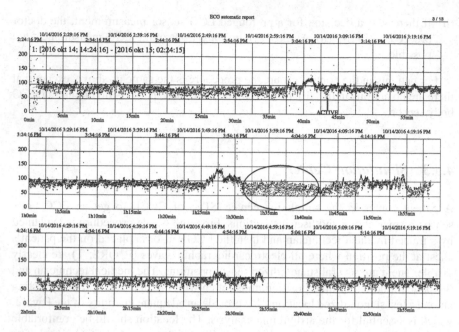

Fig. 4.1 Heart rate shown as a BPM graph obtained from an automatically generated ECG report (3 h of recording are shown in 3 lines). Each point represents a heartbeat at an instantaneous BPM

instantaneous heart rate normalized per minute, defined as $BPM = 60/(RR\ time)$, where RR is the interval between two consecutive R waves. The graphic presentation of the BPM is obtained automatically, by a computer-supported beat detector and a visual report over the whole ECG recording. There are some simple rules that can help in an initial visual examination of the ECG report:

- In sinus rhythm, especially at higher heart rates, the RR time intervals between successive beats have similar length, and consequently also the BPM, which leads to a narrow line of points in the BPM graph.
- At lower heart rates, there is often the respiratory sinus arrhythmia that broadens the BPM line.
- In the case of AF, the BPM line will be normally extremely broadened, because of non-synchronized heart activity.
- Each premature ventricular beat can be detected by a pair of points that stand out from the BPM line, the first being significantly above the BPM line and the second being significantly below the BPM line.

We found out that on one-hour BPM intervals, all common important arrhythmic evens can be identified. With a presentation of one one-hour BPM graph per line, it is possible to perform an initial examination of a long-term recording quite fast, because, e.g., 24-h of ECG fit on four A4 pages of the ECG report. In case of doubts,

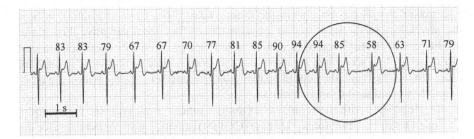

Fig. 4.2 Details from the ECG signal: sinus rhythm, because the P waves are present before each QRS complex, and unusually high HRV. The BPM goes from 94 to 58 in just 2 beats (*encircled*)

we can simply look into the original ECG measurement at that time point to see all the details of the ECG signal.

In Fig. 4.1, an example of an unusually broad BPM line is shown, even at higher heart rates. The ECG signal of about ten minutes from the encircled region, with extremely high HRV, is shown in Fig. 4.2. Visual examination of the region confirms high HRV, but still a sinus rhythm, because the P waves are clearly visible before each QRS complex. The recording is from a young male.

4.5 Long-Term ECG Data and New Knowledge

The sensor ECGs are bipolar measurements that enable a new, narrower look on the heart. In the case of several such sensors, we are able to sample the body potentials on several independent locations, which provides opportunities for new ways of ECG signal interpretation. The vast amount of ECG data that can be expected from a broad use of ECG sensors cannot be practically analyzed by visual inspection. New data analytics of the ECG Bigdata needs to be developed, substantially supported by advanced computer programs based on knowledge management and extraction. Furthermore, two proximal electrodes could provide novel answers to the old questions in electrocardiography.

The genesis of the T wave in ECG is not completely understood and is a subject of controversy. Is the T wave a result of transmural heterogeneity of repolarization or heterogeneity among different parts of the heart (apex to base) or both [13, 14]? Next, the underlying electrophysiological basis of the U wave genesis [15] has not been precisely elucidated. Several hypotheses have been proposed, e.g. delayed repolarization, mechanoelectrical interactions, transmural dispersion of repolarization, etc. The recordings from ECG sensors could contribute to the resolution of these questions.

Another uncertainty arises when we observe the cardiac rhythm. The sinus rhythm, which is the normal one, by definition originates from the sinus node in the atrium. However, in 1988, Boineau et al. demonstrated that a widely distributed atrial pacemaker complex is present in the human heart [16]. There is a question how the physiology of the heart makes these structures functional and alive throughout the life cycle. These structures are often called "ectopic focuses". A question arises: Do these regions serve as a "backup" for the sinus node function or as something else? On the one hand, they could be redundant pacemaker regions, but on the other hand, they could lead to an arrhythmia.

Beside patients with an irregular heart rhythm, other chronic patients, for example, Chronic Obstructive Pulmonary Disease (COPD) patients, are also candidates for the ECG sensor monitoring. According to the World Health Organization (WHO), the COPD is the third most frequent cause of death worldwide [17]. COPD patients are usually outpatients, except in cases of exacerbation (sudden worsening of their health status, which happens in average 1–4 times per year), for which they might be hospitalized. More than 70% of COPD–related healthcare costs are a consequence of emergencies and hospital stays for the treatment of exacerbation [18]. On the other hand, remote monitoring can reduce the frequency and severity of COPD exacerbation symptoms [19], and consequently reduce the costs.

Reports show that the primary cause of death for COPD patients is cardiac failure [20, 21]. Myocardial infarction is the co-morbidity with the greatest potential for treatment and prevention to improve the prognosis of COPD patients [20]. In general, cardiovascular diseases are the most frequent comorbidities with COPD and include the following entities: coronary artery disease, heart failure (about 30% of patients with stable COPD show some degree of heart failure), arrhythmias, and hypertension [22, 23]. It is, therefore, of the highest importance to continuously monitor cardiac electrical activity and issue alarms when dangerous events are detected. Besides, one of the signs of COPD exacerbation is respiratory rate over 25/min [24]. It is, therefore, important to measure also the respiratory rate, which is possible with no extra devices, as explained in Sect. 2.4.

A few indicative examples obtained from long-term ECG measurements are presented in the next chapter. All the cases have been obtained from volunteering users of the Savvy ECG sensor.

4.6 Sensor ECG Examples

4.6.1 Extranodal Pacemakers

An examination of an overnight sensor ECG measurement, reported previously in a paper by Avbelj [25], is presented in the following with more details. From the previous chapters, we know that a sensor ECG recording encompasses a variety of information that can be extracted from the raw sensor ECG signal. The amplitude and the morphology of the ECG waves change according to the change of the ECG sensor position relative to the heart. Using this phenomenon, the respiration rate can be derived from the ECG, as explained in Sect. 2.4. User activities can be evaluated by

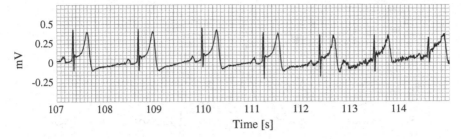

Fig. 4.3 Muscle noise in ECG is used for the detection of an effort to change the body position during the sleep. See the noise starting at the 112th second

an additional 3-D acceleration (gravity) sensor that is able to reliably measure body movements and body position changes. However, the activity can be evaluated also from the ECG signal. For example, the skeletal muscle signals (EMG) superimposed to the ECG signal are normally taken as an unwanted noise, but they can be an indicator of an activity or of an effort to change the position of the body during the sleep (see Fig. 4.3).

Further examination of the same ECG recording revealed unexpected extranodal pacemaker activity, which is usually not recognized as a normal physiological activity of the atrium. In Fig. 4.4, we see several fast changes of the heart rate during the night. The most striking event was observed around 5 AM. The heart rate increased from 48 BPM to 86 BPM in less than 15s, then quickly dropped to 55–58 BPM, and finally dropped abruptly to the value from before the episode, whose duration was 76s. It is not known what was the reason of the heart rate speed-up after the 109th second. Interestingly, the heart rate started to rise a few seconds before the appearance of the muscle noise (at the 112th from Fig. 4.3).

An abrupt change of the morphology of the P wave (compare P waves denoted by signal markers A1 and A2 in Fig. 4.4) occurred during the speed-up of the heart rate. It seems that an alternative pacemaking region starts to lead the heart rate. After the P wave morphology had been changed, it remained the same until the end of the, when the heart rate returned to the previous value. During the slowdown of the heart rate, an abrupt change in the P wave morphology occurred again at the end of the episode (see ECG signal markers B1 and B2). The shown ECG recording evidences a complex behavior of pacemaking structures in the atria. The change in the P wave morphology can be interpreted as a change in the region of the leading pacemaker. As a provocative hypothesis, we could speculate that this episode can be seen as "a training cycle" of a particular pacemaking region, which helps to preserve this region alive and functional.

It is believed that the sinus node is the origin of each heartbeat in normal cases, although there is a growing evidence for the physiological operation of extranodal pacemaker sites, which results from a widely distributed atrial pacemaker complex in the human heart [16]. In a previous study, we documented such a pattern in the process of deceleration of the heart rate during a spontaneous cardioinhibitory syncope [26].

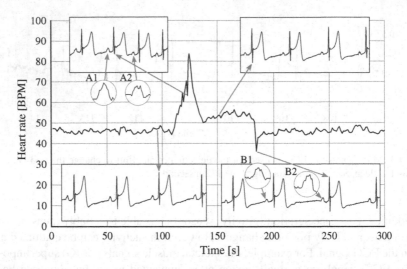

Fig. 4.4 Heart rate in an interval of 5 min around 5 AM. An abrupt change in the heart rate occurred after the 109th second and further a change in the morphology of the P wave can be seen (ECG signal markers *A1* and *A2*). During the slowdown of heart rate, an abrupt change in the morphology of the P wave occurred at the end of the episode (ECG signal markers *B1* and *B2*). This is an indication of a complex behavior of pacemaking structures in the atria

4.6.2 Atrio-Ventricular Block in an Athlete During Sleep

It is well known that the sinus node (SN) and the atrio-ventricular (AV) node are under the control of the sympathetic and parasympathetic (vagal) nervous system. The vagal branch of the system can modulate the time intervals in an ECG on a beat-by-beat basis. Higher vagal input into the SN decreases the frequency of SN depolarization, while higher vagal input into the AV node lengthens the PR interval and could even prevent the conduction of a depolarization wave from atria to ventricles—vagally mediated AV block [27].

In the following, we analyze a 24-h single-channel ECG recording with the electrodes positioned approximately at the positions of V1 and V2 of the standard 12-lead ECG. From the previous chapters, we know that in this case, the ECG represents the potential difference between V2 and V1. The ECG recording was made by a young athlete (20 years) with an ECG body sensor. The need for the measurement emerged when a missing QRS complex was noticed on the phone's screen while the athlete was sitting and playing with the ECG sensor. Figure 4.5 shows a stable length of prolonged PR intervals, which is classified as a first-degree AV block. It was published that such a block is present in 5–13% of athletes [28].

In the ECG of the same person during sleep at around 4 AM, intervals with low and high BPM variability exist. An example of a high BPM variability is shown in Fig. 4.6, where the BPM changes from 63 to 39 in just a few seconds. Note that in the intervals with high BPM variability, the PR intervals did not change in proportion to

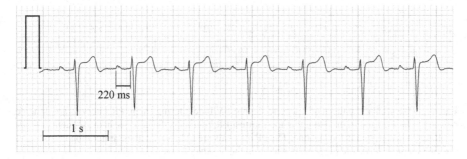

Fig. 4.5 The PR interval of a young athlete in the evening (7 PM) is constant but prolonged, indicating a first-degree AV block (PR > 200 ms). The heart rate is in a normal range of 67–70 BPM

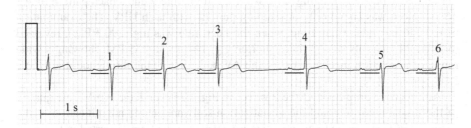

Fig. 4.6 The PR intervals do not change in proportion to the change of the RR intervals. The bars under the the PR intervals are of the same length (320 ms). The RR interval from the 3rd to the 4th QRS complex is much longer (1531 ms) than the other RR intervals, while the PR intervals of the shown beats do not differ significantly. The varying morphology of the QRS complexes is probably the influence of respiration on the differential lead vector

the RR intervals change, which indicates that different mechanisms govern the SN and AV nodes.

Quite a different situation is shown in Fig. 4.7 on the ECG of the same person at 4:39 AM. Not all atrial depolarizations are conducted to the ventricles. The conduction is blocked in a Wenckebach pattern, where successive PR intervals become longer until a block in the AV node occurs and the QRS complex is missing after the P wave. The shortest PR interval is the first one after the block. If we examine what is going on after the missing QRS complexes, we can see that in such PP intervals (indicated in Fig. 4.7 with their duration in ms: 1135, 1103 and 1047) there is a deficit of blood flow from the ventricles to the aorta and to the lungs, so that the blood pressure in the aorta falls well below the diastolic blood pressure. It could be expected that the baroreflex mechanism should speed-up the SN by lowering the vagal excitation in order to make these three PP intervals shorter. However, this was not the case, as all three PP intervals are longer than the previous ones.

The shortening of the PP intervals emerged only in the succeeding PP intervals. This is not an expected result and we have not yet found an explanation for such a behavior in the literature. It is known that such an AV block can emerge in athletes

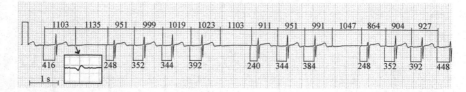

Fig. 4.7 Wenckebach pattern of a second-degree AV block during sleep. PR intervals are denoted below the ECG signal in ms. Note that the shortest PR interval is the first one in the sequence, while the longest PR interval is the last one. The PP intervals are indicated with their duration in ms above the ECG signal. A detailed P wave is shown in the zoomed frame

(type I second-degree AV block) and is most probably an expression of hypervagotonia related to physical training [27]. We noticed that the Wenckebach pattern of AV node's block was found only in sleeping periods with high HRV. The examination of the PR intervals at day-time, when the heart rate was high (90 BPM), revealed that the PR intervals were 3 times shorter, e.g. 144 ms at 4:35 PM, showing a wide range of adaptation mechanisms for the AV node delay time throughout the whole 24-h period.

Although the amplitude of the P waves in Fig. 4.7 is small ($< 50\,\mu V$), the quality of the digital recording and the visualization software enable magnification of the recorded ECG signal up to the quantization level (see the frame inserted in Fig. 4.7). In this way, the P waves and other details could be clearly seen and reproduced on the paper media. For the same reason, extensive filtering of the signal should be only an option in the post-processing phase. Therefore, we show such unfiltered signals in all figures of this chapter. It is high time that the industry qualified to produce ECG machines makes available, as a standard option, all the details of digital recordings for further analysis and research. Modern ECG machines produce excellent digital recordings, but the output is normally written only on a paper with poor resolution, which prevents detailed analysis because all details are lost. We encounter such examples in many scientific papers that offer reproductions of the ECG waveforms only from paper media with extraordinarily poor resolution.

4.6.3 Atrial Flutter During a 20-Day ECG Measurement

Finally, we present a case of a man (73 years old) with arrhythmia originating from the atria in a period of nearly 3 weeks. Again, as in the previous cases, a single-channel ECG sensor has been used with a great success. The user has reported that wearing the sensor during the 3-week period was a simple task because he had mostly forgot about wearing it.

The placement of the ECG sensor was the same as in the previous example, so that the potential difference (V2–V1) of the standard 12-lead ECG was measured. Soon after the placement of the sensor, on the first day, the ECG revealed a clear

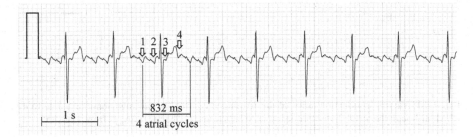

Fig. 4.8 Atrial flutter with atrial rate of 288 cycles/min (208 ms cycle period) with 4:1 conduction ratio to the ventricles. The ventricular rate is exactly 4 times lower than the atrial rate, i.e. 72 BPM

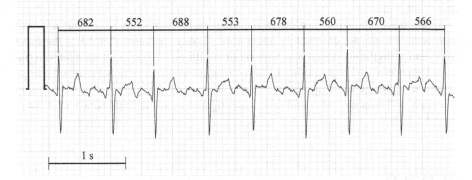

Fig. 4.9 Alternate atria-ventricle conduction. RR intervals are denoted with their duration in ms. The sum of 2 consecutive RR intervals is around 1237 ms, which produces an average ventricular rate of 97 BPM. The dominant atrial frequency is around 290 cycles/min and is not different from the situation shown in Fig. 4.8

atrial flutter pattern, shown in Fig. 4.8. If we look at the atrial waves just before the QRS complexes, we see that the atrial and the ventricular activities are coordinated, i.e., have the same phase, and that the time between the atrial waves preceding the QRS is constant. As the atrial rate is constantly at 288 cycles/min, the ventricular rate is 4 times lower.

At 6 PM of the first recording day, another atria-ventricle conduction pattern appeared, with an alternation of longer and shorter cycles (shown in Fig. 4.9). Note that the similarity of atrial waves is lost, indicating that an irregular and more complex depolarization pattern of the atria is present, although the regularity over 2 ventricular beats is still present. The only way for the autonomic system to control the ventricular rate is through a modulation of the conduction properties of the AV node.

During the night, the atrial flutter persisted, but the conduction ratio differed from that seen at day-time because of varying conduction ratios, as shown in Fig. 4.10. The latter "controlled" the average ventricular rate to a value of 49 BPM, although the atrial flutter frequency was still high (267 cycles/min). Note that each QRS complex starts nearly at the same phase with the atrial wave, just as in Fig. 4.8.

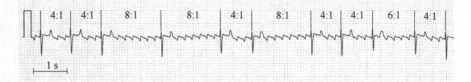

Fig. 4.10 Varying conduction ratios of the AV node "control" the average ventricular rate to 49 BPM, although the atrial flutter frequency is 267 cycles/min. The recording is from 1:30 AM

Similar situations persisted in the following days of the measurement, till the day 20, when the atrial flutter started to shift between irregular atrial waveforms of fibrillation and atrial flutter.

Even though the AF was discovered more than 100 years ago, its mechanisms and manifestation are not completely understood. Today we know that AF is the most prevalent arrhythmia, associated with other health problems and with a substantial cost. Long-term and high-quality ECG measurements can contribute to new findings in this area. We expect that other manifestations of AF, e.g. paroxismal AF or silent AF [29], will become more and more investigated by using body sensors for long-term ECG measurements.

References

1. Avbelj, V., Trobec, R., Gersak, B.: Beat-to-beat repolarisation variability in body surface electrocardiograms. Med. Biol. Eng. Comput. **41**(5), 556–560 (2003)
2. Lovric, S.S., Avbelj, V., Trobec, R., Zorman, D., Rakovec, P., Hojker, S., Gersak, B., Milcinski, M.: Sympathetic reinnervation after heart transplantation, assessed by iodine-123 metaiodobenzylguanidine imaging, and heart rate variability. Euro. J. Cardio-Thorac. Surg. **26**(4), 736–741 (2004)
3. Kalisnik, J.M., Avbelj, V., Trobec, R., Ivaskovic, D., Vidmar, G., Troise, G., Gersak, B.: Assessment of cardiac autonomic regulation and ventricular repolarization after off-pump coronary artery bypass grafting. Heart Surg. Forum **9**(3), E661–E667 (2006)
4. Kalisnik, J.M., Avbelj, V., Trobec, R., Gersak, B.: Position-dependent changes in vagal modulation after coronary artery bypass grafting. Comput. Biol. Med. **37**(10), 1404–1408 (2007)
5. Kalisnik, J.M., Avbelj, V., Trobec, R., Ivaskovic, D., Vidmar, G., Troise, G., Gersak, B.: Effects of beating-versus arrested-heart revascularization on cardiac autonomic regulation and arrhythmias. Heart Surg. Forum **10**(4), E279–E287 (2007)
6. Ksela, J., Kalisnik, J.M., Avbelj, V., Vidmar, G., Suwalski, P., Suwalski, G., Suwalski, K., Gersak, B.: Short-versus long-term ECG recordings for the assessment of non-linear heart rate variability parameters after beating heart myocardial revascularization. Comput. Biol. Med. **39**(1), 79–87 (2009)
7. Ksela, J., Suwalski, P., Kalisnik, J.M., Avbelj, V., Suwalski, G., Gersak, B.: Assessment of nonlinear heart rate dynamics after beating-heart revascularization. Heart Surg. Forum **12**(1), E10–E16 (2009)
8. Ksela, J., Kalisnik, J.M., Avbelj, V., Suwalski, P., Suwalski, G., Gersak, B.: Ventricular arrhythmic disturbances and autonomic modulation after beating-heart revascularization in patients with pulmonary normotension. Wiener klinische Wochenschrift **121**(9–10), 324–329 (2009)

9. Ksela, J., Avbelj, V., Kalisnik, J.M.: The impact of beating-heart myocardial revascularization on multifractal properties of heartbeat dynamics. Int. J. Cardiol. **177**(3), 1111–1112 (2014)
10. Ksela, J., Avbelj, V., Kalisnik, J.M.: Multifractality in heartbeat dynamics in patients undergoing beating-heart myocardial revascularization. Comput. Biol. Med. **60**, 66–73 (2015)
11. Susič, T.P., Stanič, U.: Penetration of the ICT technology to the health care primary sector— Ljubljana PILOT. In: Proceedings of Electronics and Microelectronics (MIPRO) 2016 39th Internatinal Convention Information and Communication Technology, pp. 436–441 (2016)
12. Kališnik, J.M., Susič, A.P., Semeja, A., Korošec, T., Trobec, R., Avbelj, V., Depolli, M., Stanič, U.: Mobile health monitoring pilot systems. In: Proceedings of Information Society (IS 2015), pp. 62–65 (2015)
13. Patel, C., Burke, J.F., Patel, H., Gupta, P., Kowey, P.R., Antzelevitch, C., Yan, G.-X.: Is there a significant transmural gradient in repolarization time in the intact heart? Cellular basis of the T wave: a century of controversy. Circ. Arrhythm. Electrophysiol. **2**(1), 80–88 (2009)
14. Opthof, T., Coronel, R., Janse, M.J.: Is there a significant transmural gradient in repolarization time in the intact heart?: repolarization gradients in the intact heart. Circ. Arrhythm. Electrophysiol. **2**(1), 89–96 (2009)
15. Depolli, M., Avbelj, V., Trobec, R.: Computer-simulated alternative modes of U-wave genesis. J. Cardiovasc. Electrophysiol. **19**(1), 84–89 (2008)
16. Boineau, J.P., Canavan, T.E., Schuessler, R.B., Cain, M.E., Corr, P.B., Cox, J.L.: Demonstration of a widely distributed atrial pacemaker complex in the human heart. Circulation **77**(6), 1221–1237 (1988)
17. W. H. Organisation, The top 10 causes of death (2014). http://www.who.int/mediacentre/factsheets/fs310/en/
18. Sullivan, S.D., Ramsey, S.D., Lee, T.A.: The economic burden of COPD. Chest **117**(2, Supplement), 5S–9S (2000)
19. Cordova, F.C., Ciccolella, D., Grabianowski, C., Gaughan, J., Brennan, K., Goldstein, F., Jacobs, M.R., Criner, G.J.: A telemedicine-based intervention reduces the frequency and severity of COPD exacerbation symptoms: a randomized controlled trial. Telemed. e-Health **22**(2), 114–122 (2015)
20. Sode, B.F., Dahl, M., Nordestgaard, B.G.: Myocardial infarction and other co-morbidities in patients with chronic obstructive pulmonary disease: a Danish Nationwide Study of 7.4 million individuals. Euro. Heart J. **32**(19), 2365–2375 (2011)
21. Zvezdin, B., Milutinov, S., Kojicic, M., Hadnadjev, M., Hromis, S., Markovic, M., Gajic, O.: A postmortem analysis of major causes of early death in patients. Chest **136**(2), 376–380 (2009)
22. Vestbo, J., Hurd, S.S., Agustí, A.G., Jones, P.W., Vogelmeier, C., Anzueto, A., Barnes, P.J., Fabbri, L.M., Martinez, F.J., Nishimura, M., Stockley, R.A., Sin, D.D., Rodriguez-Roisin, R.: Global strategy for the diagnosis, management, and prevention of chronic obstructive pulmonary disease GOLD executive summary. Am. J. Respir. Crit. Care Med. **187**(4), 347–365 (2013)
23. Falk, J.A., Kadiev, S., Criner, G.J., Scharf, S.M., Minai, O.A., Diaz, P.: Cardiac disease in chronic obstructive pulmonary disease. Proc. Am. Thorac. Soc. **5**(4), 543–548 (2008)
24. Siafakas, N.M., Vermeire, P., Pride, N.B., Paoletti, P., Gibson, J., Howard, P., Yernault, J.C., Decramer, M., Higenbottam, T., Postma, D.S., Rees, J.: Optimal assessment and management of chronic obstructive pulmonary disease (COPD). Euro. Respir. J. **8**(8), 1398–1420 (1995)
25. Avbelj, V.: Extranodal pacemaker activity during sleep—a case study of wireless ECG sensor data. In: Proceedings of Electronics and Microelectronics (MIPRO) 2015 38th International Convention Information and Communication Technology, pp. 370–372 (2015)
26. Avbelj, V., Trobec, R.: A closer look at electrocardiographic p waves before and during spontaneous cardioinhibitory syncope. Int. J. Cardiol. **166**(3), e59–e61 (2013)
27. Barold, S.S., Herweg, B.: Second-degree atrioventricular block revisited. Herzschrittmacherther Elektrophysiol. **23**(4), 296–304 (2012)
28. Prakash, K., Sharma, S.: Interpretation of the Electrocardiogram in Athletes. Can. J. Cardiol. **32**(4), 438–451 (2016)
29. Dilaveris, P.E., Kennedy, H.L.: Silent atrial fibrillation: epidemiology, diagnosis, and clinical impact. Clin. Cardiol. 1–6 (2017)

Chapter 5
Lead Theory of Differential Leads and Synthesis of the Standard 12-Lead ECG

Abstract In this chapter, the lead theory of differential leads is presented. A differential lead is an ECG lead obtained from two closely positioned electrodes on the body surface. It can be measured with an ECG body sensor. The theoretical background is needed to gain a formal and intuitive understanding of what is measured with differential leads, as well as to elaborate how the standard 12-lead ECG can be synthesized from three differential leads. The 12-lead ECG synthesis is based on the dipole volume source model. After introducing the dipole model, the Burger's equation is derived and the concept of lead vector defined. We describe how to derive lead vectors from known heart vector and, vice versa, how to obtain the heart vector from known lead vectors. Then, the concepts of image surface and lead field are introduced, followed with a description of the lead field of a differential lead. Next, the theory and methods for ECG leads synthesis from differential leads is presented. The chapter concludes with a discussion on the evaluation and personalization of the synthesis.

5.1 Preconditions

Depending on the purpose, different assumptions will be made throughout this chapter regarding the characteristics of the volume source and the volume conductor. Common assumptions of the lead theory are that *a human body is a quasi-static and linear physical system.*

Cardiac electrical sources are a consequence of the electrical activity of the myocardium cell membranes, i.e., of ion flows through the membranes. Since these activities vary with time (different cells and different numbers of cells are depolarized or repolarized), the resulting electrical potential field established in the volume conductor is time-varying. The quasi-static assumption states that all the fields: those in the volume source, i.e. in the heart, and those in the volume conductor, i.e. in the body, are synchronous, as if the sources were static. In other words, at any time instant, the electrical field throughout the body, or the resulting potential field at the body surface, will be a consequence of a stationary source at the same instant. A consequence of the quasi-static conditions is that from the distribution of sources at

© The Author(s) 2018   77
R. Trobec et al., *Body Sensors and Electrocardiography*, SpringerBriefs
in Applied Sciences and Technology, DOI 10.1007/978-3-319-59340-1_5

a given time instant, the corresponding extra-cardiac field can be determined without any regard to the source distribution in the past.

For the *quasi-static* conditions to be met, the following should be satisfied [3]:

1. negligible propagation effect, i.e., negligible time required for the propagation of changes in the source to any field point,
2. negligible capacitive effect,
3. negligible inductive effect.

By using the electrical properties of biological materials previously reported by Rush et al. [1] and Schwan and Kay [2], Plonsey and Heppner [3] showed that the above conditions are met for frequencies up to 1 kHz and for distances up to 1 m.

For an intuitive justification and understanding of the quasi-static nature of the bioelectrical phenomena, it is helpful to consider the rate of change of the involved fields, which is not fast enough to prevent the consequential potential field on the body surface from being observed at the moment when the change of the source field occurs.

The *linearity* of the system means that whenever a source is increased by a factor, the resulting potential field will be increased by the same factor. The linearity also means that a linear combination of sources produces a linear combination of responses that would have been caused by each source individually. This property of linear systems is also called *the principle of superposition* or the superposition property.

In summary, the resulting potential field and currents through the volume conductor at any time instant depend only on the sources at that instant and obey the principle of superposition.

5.2   Dipole as a Volume Source Model

An important task in electrocardiography is to solve the inverse problem, i.e., to determine or estimate the electrical sources in the heart that resulted in a measured potential distribution on the body surface (or some other describable surface) at each instant of time. It is, however, obvious that for any three-dimensional potential distribution, there is an infinite number of electrical cardiac sources that can induce it [4–6]. This is because one can always add sources that generate no field or a field below the noise level.

After we have established that there is no unique mapping between body surface potentials and electrical sources in the heart, it is evident that the inverse problem can be solved only if a model of the volume source is assumed. To solve the inverse problem then means to determine the value of the parameters describing the assumed model. Please note that the solution of the inverse problem is always just a model, and consequently does not exist in reality.

There are different possible models for the volume source, e.g. dipole, quadrupole, octapole, and so on, and finally multipole. A model that generates the same potentials on the body surface as the actual primary source is called *equivalent source* or *equivalent generator*. The multipole is an example of such a model [6]. We will, however, concentrate on the dipole model, since it is the central model used in ECG synthesis theory. Furthermore, it will be shown that cardiac electrical activity on the body surface can be predominately explained by the dipole volume source model.

Geselowitz has shown in [6] that the heart dipole can be expressed in terms of impressed currents as:

$$\vec{p}_H = \int_{V_H} \vec{J}^i dV - \sum_j \int_{S_j} (\sigma' - \sigma'') \phi d\vec{S}_j, \tag{5.1}$$

where V_H is the heart volume, $\vec{J}^i$ is the impressed current density associated with the active behavior of the cell membranes, $d\vec{S}_j$ is a differential element of the surface S_j that separates regions of conductivity σ' and σ'', and ϕ is the potential at $d\vec{S}_j$. Note that $d\vec{S}_j$ is a vector surface element that is by convention directed from the σ' region towards the σ'' region. The equation provides an arbitrary number of surfaces j that separate regions of different conductivities. The major discontinuities in conductivity are inner and outer surfaces of the heart, i.e., the surface between the myocardium and the intracavitary blood mass, and the surface between the myocardium and the lungs.

For a homogeneous conductor, $\sigma' = \sigma'' = \sigma$ applies, so that the previous Eq. 5.1 reduces to:

$$\vec{p}_H = \int_{V_H} \vec{J}^i dV, \tag{5.2}$$

which indicates that $\vec{J}^i$ is a dipole moment per unit volume (i.e., the dipole density) and $\vec{J}^i dV$ is a single dipole source component of the heart dipole $\vec{p}_H$. Therefore, the heart vector can be considered as a sum of all the elementary dipole contributions throughout the entire volume of the heart V_H. Note that $\vec{J}^i$ changes in time, because the heart electrical activity is different in different time moments. Consequently, the vector $\vec{p}_H$ changes its magnitude, direction and location through time. Note that the terms "heart dipole" and "heart vector" are used as synonyms. We denote the exact heart vector $\vec{p}_H$ with subscript H to distinguish it from all the other fictitious dipoles used to model a heart, which are also commonly called heart vectors.

The heart dipole, as expressed by Eq. 5.1, is only the first term of the possible multipole expansion that provides a complete description of the equivalent generator [6]. An obvious, but important consequence is that the heart dipole does not produce the same potential distribution on the body surface as the real heart source or an equivalent generator. Still, as we are going to see in Sect. 5.7.1, there is a lot of evidence that the heart is predominately a dipolar source. Even though the recording sites can be close to the heart, depending on the employed lead system, additional justification for considering the heart as a dipole comes from the fact that any complex source with a zero net current can be approximated by a dipole, with an improvement in approximation as the observation distance becomes greater than the largest dimension of the source [7]. The condition of net current, i.e., the algebraic sum of currents being equal to zero, is satisfied by the heart since no net charge is generated at any instant.

The heart dipole $\vec{p}_H$ has a location that is time-dependent. As the observation distance from the heart increases, the dislocation of $\vec{p}_H$ from the heart centroid becomes more and more negligible. Therefore, the vector $\vec{p}_H$ is sometimes assumed to be at the center of the heart region, although its position is time-dependent. The source model which assumes a dipole with a fixed location and variable orientation and magnitude is called *fixed dipole model*. On the other hand, the source model which assumes not only varying orientation and magnitude, but also varying location for a single dipole, is called *moving dipole model*. Depending on the purpose, the location of the heart dipole can be relevant or irrelevant. It is important to note that to uniquely describe a fixed dipole, its three Cartesian coordinates (or in spherical coordinates: magnitude and two direction angles) are necessary. For describing a moving dipole, however, six independent variables are necessary: three for describing the dipole vector and three for describing the dislocation vector.

5.3 Lead Vector

Einthoven's classical lead theory [8, 9] is based on the assumption that the human body is a part of a spherical or an infinitive homogeneous conductor, in which the heart electrical sources are represented by a single, two-dimensional time-varying dipole that has a fixed location in the frontal plane of the human body, at the center of the homogeneous sphere. Burger and van Milaan developed a more precise lead theory, referred to as the volume-conductor theory [10, 11], by assuming that the human body is a three-dimensional, bounded, irregularly shaped and inhomogeneous volume conductor. Their lead theory also relies on the fixed dipole hypothesis. According to it, the potentials anywhere on the body surface can be derived by projecting the heart dipole on directions in three dimensional space called lead vectors.

The lead vector is a concept that provides ECG leads with a formal spatial interpretation. It is a time-invariant vector in space describing the direction in which a certain lead monitors the cardiac electrical activity. The length of the lead vector determines the lead measurement sensitivity. Figure 5.1 shows the Einthoven triangle of limb lead vectors obtained under Einthoven's assumptions.

The Burger's equation formally relates the voltage on a given lead to its lead vector:

$$L = \vec{L} \cdot \vec{p}, \tag{5.3}$$

where $\vec{p}$ is a dipole describing the cardiac electrical activity, not necessarily equal to $\vec{p}_H$. For instance, $\vec{p}$ can be an artificial dipole placed in a volume conductor model for experimental purposes.

As an example of the Burger's equation application, consider the case where two points determining a bipolar lead are on the left and the right arms (Fig. 5.1).

Fig. 5.1 Einthoven triangle. All the lead vectors lie in the frontal plane of the human body, defined by the x-y coordinate system vectors. The projections of the heart vector $\vec{p_H}$ on the sides of the triangle are equal to the scalar product of the heart vector and the normalized lead vectors (Burger's equation)

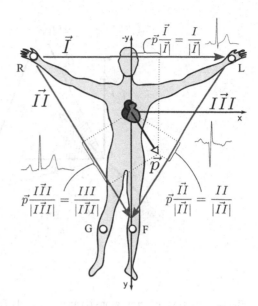

According to the Burger's equation 5.3, the measured voltage of the bipolar lead is: $I = \vec{I} \cdot \vec{p}$.

The Burger's equation is in fact the definition of the lead vector—the vector that, when multiplied by the dipole representing the heart, provides the measured lead voltage. The Burger's equation is also a statement that such a vector exists for every choice of the vector $\vec{p}$. The question remains how to obtain the lead vector for a specific lead. From the Burger's equation, it is obvious that to calculate $\vec{L}$, one needs to know the voltage measured on a lead and the vector $\vec{p}$. Normally, one would employ a model of the volume conductor inside which a dipole is energized and measure potentials on the model's surface. More details on the procedure for obtaining lead vectors are provided in Sect. 5.3.2.

For the scalar product $\vec{L} \cdot \vec{p}$ to be evaluated by $L = |\vec{L}| \cdot |\vec{p}| \cdot \cos(\theta)$, where θ is the angle between the vectors, the location of $\vec{p}$ and $\vec{L}$ relative to each other is irrelevant. Hence, the vectors $\vec{L}$ and $\vec{p}$ can be placed at the origin of an arbitrary coordinate system. The system is normally chosen to have origin at the position of the negative pole of $\vec{p}$ (see Fig. 5.2). The rationale for this choice comes from the fact that the orientation and length of each lead vectors $\vec{L}$ depends on the locations of the corresponding vector $\vec{p}$ (will be explained in Sect. 5.5). It is, therefore, convenient to give each vector $\vec{p}$ and the corresponding vector $\vec{L}$ a common starting point.

The Burger's equation was derived under the assumption that the inhomogeneous and irregularly shaped human body is a linear physical system (Sect. 5.1). Besides the location of the vector $\vec{p}$, the vector $\vec{L}$ also reflects the inhomogeneities and the shape of the volume conductor, when deriving the lead voltage from a known $\vec{p}$. More details on this are provided in Sect. 5.5.

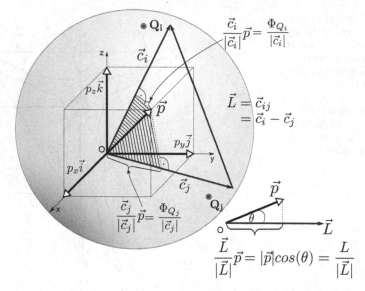

Fig. 5.2 Heart vector projections on axes and leads. $\vec{c}_i$ and $\vec{c}_j$ are the unipolar lead vectors for the points Q_i and Q_j, respectively, whereas $\vec{L}$ is the bipolar lead vector. The projection of the heart vector on a lead vector, multiplied by the length of the lead vector, is the lead voltage. The medium (volume source and volume conductor) is conductive, linear, and inhomogeneous

5.3.1   The Burger's Equation

A dipole is a pair of a current source and a current sink of the same current strength I_d and separated by a small displacement d. The mathematical definition of a dipole requires $d \rightarrow 0$, $I_d \rightarrow \infty$, with $p = I_d \cdot d$ remaining finite. The quantity p is the moment or magnitude of the dipole. The dipole is a vector $\vec{p}$ with magnitude p and direction from the negative source (sink) towards the positive source [12].

It is worth noting that "perfect" mathematical dipoles, i.e., dipoles with $d \rightarrow 0$, do not exist in electrophysiology. The "real" physical dipoles, like those formed on cell membranes, have a displacement greater than zero (e.g. membrane thicknesses). Still, mathematical dipoles are often used as an approximation for physical dipoles, for practical reasons, because the mathematical dipoles are described with concise formulas. The approximation of physical dipoles as mathematical dipoles holds for $d/r < 0.1$, where r is the displacement from the dipole, i.e., if the observation distance is at least ten times larger than the displacement of the monopoles forming the dipole [13].

Let us assume a three-dimensional coordinate system $(\vec{i}, \vec{j}, \vec{k})$ with a reference potential located at its origin. Let $\phi_Q^{\vec{i}}$ be the potential at an arbitrary point Q caused by the unit dipole $\vec{i}$. By using the linearity assumption, the potential $\phi_Q^{p_x \vec{i}}$ corresponding to the dipole $p_x \vec{i}$ of an arbitrary magnitude p_x is:

$$\phi_Q^{p_x \vec{i}} = \phi_Q^{\vec{i}} \cdot p_x. \tag{5.4}$$

An analogous expression holds for the dipoles in the $\vec{j}$ and $\vec{k}$ directions. The linearity assumption ensures the maintenance of the principle of superposition, which states that an electrical field arising from several sources is the sum of the fields that would be present if each source acted separately. The dipole in three orthogonal components is:

$$\vec{p} = p_x \vec{i} + p_y \vec{j} + p_z \vec{k}. \tag{5.5}$$

Using the principle of superposition, the potential at the point Q, caused by the dipole $\vec{p}$ at the origin of the coordinate system, is:

$$\phi_Q^{\vec{p}} = \phi_Q^{\vec{i}} p_x + \phi_Q^{\vec{j}} p_y + \phi_Q^{\vec{z}} p_z. \tag{5.6}$$

If components $\phi_Q^{\vec{i}}$, $\phi_Q^{\vec{j}}$ and $\phi_Q^{\vec{k}}$ are interpreted as the components of a vector $\vec{c}$, Eq. 5.6 can be written as:

$$\phi_Q^{\vec{p}} = \vec{c} \cdot \vec{p}. \tag{5.7}$$

The vector $\vec{c} = (\phi_Q^{\vec{i}}, \phi_Q^{\vec{j}}, \phi_Q^{\vec{k}})$ is called *lead vector of a unipolar lead*. In this case, the lead is determined by the potential at the point Q and the zero potential at the origin of the coordinate system, but in general, the zero reference potential can be any local or remote reference point.

A bipolar lead whose electrodes are at points Q_i and Q_j measures the potential difference L between the two points:

$$V_{Q_1 Q_2} = L = \phi_{Q_i}^{\vec{p}} - \phi_{Q_j}^{\vec{p}}. \tag{5.8}$$

In the following, we will use L instead of $V_{Q_1 Q_2}$ to designate a lead voltage in situations not requiring reference to the names of the points Q_1 and Q_2 that determine the lead. By substituting $\phi_{Q_i}^{\vec{p}}$ and $\phi_{Q_j}^{\vec{p}}$ according to Eq. 5.7, in Eq. 5.8, we get the Burger's equation:

$$L = \vec{c}_i \vec{p} - \vec{c}_j \vec{p} = \vec{c}_{ij} \cdot \vec{p} = \vec{L} \cdot \vec{p} = |\vec{L}| \cdot |\vec{p}| \cdot \cos(\theta), \tag{5.9}$$

where $\vec{c}_i$ and $\vec{c}_j$ are unipolar lead vectors for the points Q_i and Q_j, $\vec{L} = \vec{c}_{ij} = \vec{c}_i - \vec{c}_j$ is *the bipolar lead vector*, and θ is the angle between $\vec{L}$ and $\vec{p}$.

From Eq. 5.9, it follows that for a normalized lead vector, i.e. for $|\vec{L}| = 1$, the lead voltage L is $|\vec{p}| \cdot \cos(\theta)$—the projection of the heart vector on the lead vector. The same holds for the unipolar lead vector from Eq. 5.7. This is why a lead vector can be interpreted as a spatial direction in which the cardiac electrical activity is monitored. It follows from Eq. 5.9 that the lead voltage L is obtained by multiplying the heart vector's projection with the length of the lead vector $|\vec{L}|$. Consequently, a longer $\vec{L}$ implies a higher measured voltage. For this reason, the length of a lead vector $|\vec{L}|$ is also called *the lead sensitivity*. Alternatively, a lead vector can be thought of as a sensitivity vector with the length representing the magnitude of the lead sensitivity, whereas the direction is the direction of the lead sensitivity.

The voltage on the left side of the Burger's equation is the only directly measurable entity in living subjects. Therefore, to have a control over $\vec{p}$, a model is usually used. Then, if we know the heart vector $\vec{p}$, the Burger's equation can be applied to determine the lead vector. The Burger's equation is used also in the opposite direction: to determine $\vec{p}$ from known lead vectors. In the continuation, we will show that three lead vectors are needed for this purpose.

5.3.2 Deriving the Lead Vectors from a Known Heart Vector

Equation 5.6 can be used to experimentally find a lead vector for an arbitrary point Q on a body surface by using a mathematical or a physical torso model. The lead vector is found by energizing unit dipoles in the model's heart region along the x, y, and z axes in sequence, and measuring the potential at the point Q for each dipole. For example, if the unit dipole is oriented in the x direction, then $p_y = p_z = 0$. From Eq. 5.6, it follows that $\phi_Q^{\vec{i}} = \phi_Q^{\vec{p}}$. Since $\phi_Q^{\vec{p}}$ is the measured potential, the first element of the vector $\vec{c}$ is determined.

It is important to note that the lead vectors are not derived (and not even defined—see Eq. 5.3) by using real heart electrical sources (like, for instance, an equivalent dipole defined by Eq. 5.2) and a real volume conductor, but by experimentally placing a dipole on a fixed location in a model of a volume conductor. The more the fixed dipole is a realistic model of the source (see Sect. 5.7.1), and the more the model of the volume conductor is realistic and appropriate for each person, the more the calculated lead vectors are reliable representations of the corresponding leads' observational directions and sensitivities. Since the use of the models is in practice the only way for determining the lead vectors, it can be said that a lead vector is a vector in space, which when multiplied by a dipole source, results in a corresponding measured potential on the surface of the employed volume conductor model.

Even though lead vectors for individual $\vec{p_H}$ defined by Eq. 5.1 cannot be precisely determined in practice, they do exist in theory, since the Burger's equation states that there is always a vector $\vec{L}$ on which one vector $\vec{p}$ can be projected to produce the measured voltage. Even if we consider the $\vec{p_H}$ location as time-dependent, then for each moment in time, there is still a $\vec{L}$ that when multiplied by $\vec{p_H}$ would produce the measured voltage. Nevertheless, $\vec{L}$ is by definition time-invariant and defined for a fixed location dipole.

5.3.3 Deriving the Heart Vector from Known Lead Vectors

A dipole $\vec{p}$ describing a heart, as any other vector in space, at each instant in time has three components in Cartesian coordinates (see Eq. 5.5). To calculate the three components, one needs a system of three equations with the three components as the only unknowns. We write three Burger's equations for the three leads:

$$L(i) = \vec{L}(i) \cdot \vec{p}, \; i = 1, 2, 3, \qquad (5.10)$$

where i indexes the leads. If the three lead vectors $\vec{L}(i)$ are known a priory and if we can measure voltages on the three leads $L(i)$, then we can solve the system of Eq. 5.10 for the three components of the vector $\vec{p}$. Note that if the lead voltages are measured on a real person, but the lead vectors were previously determined by using a model (as described in Sect. 5.3.2), this procedure, in the absence of noise, results in $\vec{p}$ that, if inserted in the same model, would produce voltages equal to the voltages measured on the person. Consequently, the obtained heart vector is not equal to the heart vector defined by Eq. 5.1 and is only an estimate of it. Additionally, the vector $\vec{p}_H$ defined by Eq. 5.1 is a moving dipole, whereas the obtained vector $\vec{p}$ is fixed. In conclusion, any three independent leads suffice for an accurate representation of a fixed-location dipole, which is an estimate of the heart vector.

5.4 Image Surface

According to the procedure described in Sect. 5.3.3, the cardiac electrical activity can be described by measuring the potentials on leads with known lead vectors. It is therefore desirable to know the unipolar lead vectors for any point on a body surface.

The concept of determining lead vectors described in Sect. 5.3.2 can be applied at an arbitrary number of points on a model surface. The tips of the acquired unipolar lead vectors determine the surface known as *the image surface* or image space. Since it consists of lead vectors, an image surface can be interpreted as an alternative, imaginary torso, in which lines connecting two points represent the true monitored spatial directions of the cardiac electrical activity. The deviation of each lead vector's direction from the direction defined by the line connecting the lead's electrode positions on the body surface can be regarded as a measure of the electrical distortion of the dipole behavior as seen on the body surface [14].

The concept of image surface was introduced by Burger and van Milaan [15], but its first experimental determination was performed by Frank [16]. As a collection of lead vectors, the image surface depends on the location of the dipole and the characteristics of the volume conductor. Consequently, image surfaces are different for each person. The image surfaces are practically obtained by using physical models which are designed to be representative for all people or for a particular population.

Among all existing image surfaces, the Frank image surface, published in [16], is the one most often used in the subsequent research. Frank constructed a tank model having a thorax form, oriented it upside-down, and filled it with a salt solution. A dipole was fixed in the center of the model region, which Frank assumed to be "occupied in life by the ventricular mass during very deep inspiration". The frontal-view-triangle part of the Frank image surface can be seen to depart significantly from the equilateral Einthoven triangle, i.e., the limb lead vectors in the Frank image space are different from the Einthoven triangle lead vectors. This is because the Frank's model is not spherical, whereas the Einthoven's model is spherical, even though both models are homogeneous. For a complete specification of the Frank image surface, the reader is referred to [16].

Frank also stated that the influence of the dipole location on the lead vectors is more pronounced than the influence of the torso's shape and the inhomogeneities introduced into the model [4]. More recent image surface studies were made on computer models. Computer models make it easier to include more detailed inhomogeneities, such as intracavitary blood masses and muscle layers, as well as to investigate the influence of the dipole location on the image surface [17]. The research on computer models did not invalidate Frank's observations.

5.5 Lead Field

A lead field is a vector field consisted of lead vectors obtained for different locations of a dipole, by keeping the lead measurement points fixed. Each lead vector is placed at the position of the dipole for which it is derived. The lead field approach is opposite to the image surface approach, in which the dipole position is kept constant, while the measurement point positions are varied. We use the notation $\vec{L}(x, y, y)$ to designate a lead vector field, and $\vec{L}$ to designate a single lead vector. Given the vector field $\vec{L}(x, y, y)$, we can extend the Burger's equation 5.3 and write:

$$L = \vec{L}(x, y, y) \cdot \vec{p}(x, y, y). \tag{5.11}$$

This equations states that the measured voltage for a lead is a product of a dipole $\vec{p}$ describing the heart and the element of the lead's vector field $\vec{L}(x, y, y)$ at the same location as $\vec{p}$.

To determine the lead field for a pair of positions on the body surface, one needs to calculate lead vectors for every dipole position in a model, using the procedure described in Sect. 5.3.2. In practice, that is possible only for a finite number of dipole positions. Fortunately, there is another way of describing a lead field. The alternative approach is based on *the electromagnetic reciprocity theorem*, which states roughly the following: The relationship between a current and the resulting electric field is unchanged if one interchanges the points where the current is placed and where the field is measured. In other words, if the current source and voltmeter positions are swapped, the voltmeter reading will not be altered.

Let there be an approximate dipole formed by a point source I_d and a point sink $-I_d$ at a very small distance d in an arbitrarily shaped volume conductor. This dipole can be a heart vector $\vec{p}_H$:

$$\vec{p}_H = I_d \vec{d}. \tag{5.12}$$

Let ϕ' be the potential field of $\vec{p}_H$. Then, the voltage between the points Q_1 and Q_2 is (panel A in Fig. 5.3):

$$V_{Q_1 Q_2} = \phi'(\vec{r}_{Q_1}) - \phi'(\vec{r}_{Q_2}). \tag{5.13}$$

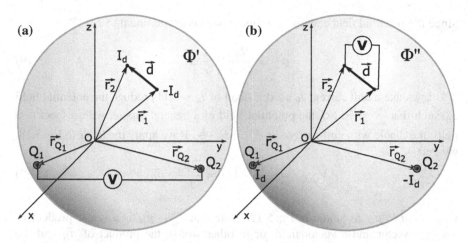

Fig. 5.3 The application of the reciprocity theorem: before and after swapping the positions of the source (I_d) and the voltmeter (V), as shown on the panels (**a**) and (**b**), the voltmeter will measure the same voltage

By applying the Burger's equation 5.3, we can also write:

$$V_{Q_1 Q_2} = L = \vec{p}_H \cdot \vec{L}_{Q_1 Q_2}, \tag{5.14}$$

where $\vec{L}_{Q_1 Q_2}$ is the lead vector for the measured voltage $V_{Q_1 Q_2} = L$.

If we swap the positions of the current source and the voltmeter (panel B in Fig. 5.3), the reciprocity theorem states that:

$$V_{Q_1 Q_2} = \phi''(\vec{r}_2) - \phi''(\vec{r}_1), \tag{5.15}$$

where ϕ'' is the potential field of the point source I_d and the point sink $-I_d$ placed at Q_1 and Q_2, respectively.

Since d is assumed to be small, to obtain $\phi''(\vec{r}_2)$, we can write the Taylor expansion for ϕ'' at $\vec{r}_1$ by including only the linear term:

$$\phi''(\vec{r}_2) = \phi''(\vec{r}_1) + \left.\frac{\partial \phi''}{\partial d}\right|_{\vec{r}_1} \cdot d. \tag{5.16}$$

Since the directional derivative (the second element on the right side of Eq. 5.16) is the same as the gradient multiplied by the unit vector in that direction, it follows:

$$\phi''(\vec{r}_2) = \phi''(\vec{r}_1) + \nabla\phi'' \cdot d \cdot \vec{a}_d = \phi''(\vec{r}_1) + \nabla\phi'' \cdot \vec{d}, \tag{5.17}$$

where $\vec{a}_d$ is the unit vector in the direction $\vec{d}$. By inserting Eq. 5.17 in Eq. 5.15, we obtain:

$$V_{Q_1 Q_2} = \nabla\phi'' \cdot \vec{d}. \tag{5.18}$$

Since the potential field caused by a dipole (ϕ_D) is proportional to I_d [13]:

$$\phi_D = \frac{I_d}{4\pi\sigma} \nabla(\frac{1}{r})\vec{d}, \qquad (5.19)$$

it follows that a unit current I_0 used instead of I_d would produce the potential field ϕ_0'' such that $\frac{\phi_0''}{\phi''} = \frac{I_0}{I_d}$. So, the potential field of a general dipole, with respect to a field of a dipole with unit current, is $\phi'' = \phi_0'' \cdot \frac{I_d}{I_0}$. If we apply the latter to Eq. 5.18, we get:

$$V_{Q_1 Q_2} = \frac{\nabla\phi_0''}{I_0} \cdot I_d\vec{d} = \frac{\nabla\phi_0''}{I_0} \cdot \vec{p}_H, \qquad (5.20)$$

where $I_d\vec{d} = \vec{p}_H$ as stated in Eq. 5.12. Note that $\frac{\nabla\phi_0''}{I_0} \cdot \vec{p}_H$ is a scalar product of a single vector and a vector field, or in other words, the product of $\vec{p}_H$ and the corresponding vector at the same position in $\nabla\phi_0''$. By comparing Eqs. 5.20 and 5.14, it is obvious that:

$$\vec{L}_{Q_1 Q_2}(x, y, z) = \frac{\nabla\phi_0''}{I_0}, \qquad (5.21)$$

where $\vec{L}_{Q_1 Q_2}(x, y, z)$ is the lead field for the lead defined by the points Q_1 and Q_2. $\vec{L}_{Q_1 Q_2}(x, y, z)$ is used to express that it refers to a vector field, compared to $\vec{L}_{Q_1 Q_2}$, which is a single vector.

Equation 5.21 states that a lead field is equal to the gradient of the potential field caused by a pair of a unit current source and a sink placed at the lead's electrodes positions. For an intuitive representation of a lead field, it is helpful to take into account that the current density in the volume conductor is directly proportional to the gradient of the potential $\vec{J}_0^L = -\sigma\nabla\phi_0''$. If we apply this fact to Eq. 5.21, we get:

$$\vec{L}_{Q_1 Q_2}(x, y, z) = \frac{\nabla\phi_0''}{I_0} = \frac{-\vec{J}_0^L}{I_0\sigma}, \qquad (5.22)$$

where $\vec{J}_0^L = \vec{J}_0^L(x, y, z)$ denotes the current density due to unit reciprocal current. Hence, the lead field structure for the lead defined by two electrodes is equivalent to the structure of the current density between the same two electrodes, but respecting that the current and the potential gradient have opposite directions (see Fig. 5.4).

If we consider the heart vector to be the sum of all the elementary dipole contributions (Eq. 5.2), we may apply the superposition principle on Eq. 5.20, to obtain:

$$V_{Q_1 Q_2} = L = \int \frac{\nabla\phi_0''}{I_0} \cdot \vec{J}^i dV = \frac{1}{I_0} \int \left(\frac{-\vec{J}_0^L}{\sigma}\right) \cdot \vec{J}^i dV, \qquad (5.23)$$

where σ is the conductivity distribution through the heart volume, which is in general a function of position and time: $\sigma = \sigma(x, y, z, t)$, and $\vec{J}^i$ is the volume

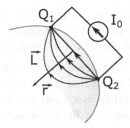

Fig. 5.4 The lead field of a differential lead. The *lines* with *arrows* within the volume conductor (*gray circle*) represent the lead field $\vec{L}$. The lead field is proportional to the current flow field arising from a unit current introduced at Q_1 and removed at Q_2, and has the opposite direction. The bowing of the field increases with r, whereas the field magnitude (i.e., the current strength) decreases with r^3

source impressed current vector field, which also depends on position and time: $\vec{J}^i = \vec{J}^i(x, y, z, t)$. If σ is constant, we can move $\frac{1}{\sigma}$ out of the integral and obtain:

$$V_{Q_1 Q_2} = \frac{-1}{I_0 \sigma} \int \vec{J}_0^L \cdot \vec{J}^i dV. \tag{5.24}$$

Equations 5.23 and 5.24 show that each element dV of the volume source contributes to the lead voltage with a component equal to the scalar product of the lead field current density at dV and the volume source impressed current element, divided by the conductivity at the same spatial element dV. In other words, the lead voltage is a weighted sum of contributing sources with weights $\nabla \phi_0'' = (\frac{-\vec{J}_0^L}{\sigma})$. This justifies the interpretation of the lead field as *the lead sensitivity distribution*, as its role in obtaining the lead voltage is to weight each source element $\vec{J}^i$. A larger magnitude of $\vec{J}_0^L$ at dV and a smaller angle between $\vec{J}^i$ and $\vec{J}_0^L$ at dV result in a larger contribution of $\vec{J}^i$ at dV to the measured voltage.

Recall that we described (Sect. 5.3.1) the lead vector as the sensitivity vector for one location of a dipole. The lead field is an extension of the lead vector concept for all locations of the dipole. Consequently, one lead vector, obtained for one location of the dipole, is an element of the lead field obtained by using the same model (recall that the lead vectors are always derived by using a model—Sect. 5.3.2). Multiplying $\vec{p}_H$ by its lead vector (Eq. 5.20), and multiplying each $\vec{J}^i dV$ by its lead vector and then summing the products for all dVs (Eq. 5.23), is equivalent in terms of producing the same voltage $V_{Q_1 Q_2}$ (Eqs. 5.20 and 5.23 have the same $V_{Q_1 Q_2}$ on the left). According to Eq. 5.20, $V_{Q_1 Q_2}$ is caused by $\vec{p}_H$. The real distribution of sources $\vec{J}^i$ produces a voltage different from $V_{Q_1 Q_2}$, because $\vec{p}_H$ is not an equivalent generator (as already stated in Sect. 5.2). Therefore, Eq. 5.23 should be considered as just another way of expressing Eq. 5.20.

It follows from Eq. 5.22 that the lead field will never be homogeneous in real situations, because the current field through a volume conductor is in general never homogeneous: it changes direction, and is weaker further away from the current source, as the same current passes through a larger surface. Furthermore, since σ is also a function of position and is in general different for different volume conductors, it follows that the lead field $\frac{-\vec{J}_0^L}{\sigma}$ is different for different lead measurement locations, and different shapes and conduction characteristics of the volume conductor. This is the justification for the important assertions we made in Sect. 5.3 about the lead vector: it depends on the location of the dipole, on the locations of the lead electrodes, and on the electrical characteristics and the shape of the volume conductor, but not on the magnitude or the direction of the dipole.

A special and unrealistic case is a homogeneous volume source and a constant lead field $\vec{J}_0^L = \vec{J}_C$, which weights all elementary dipoles $\vec{J}^i dV$ equally. If we rewrite Eq. 5.20 by substituting $\frac{\nabla \phi_0''}{I_0}$ with $\frac{-\vec{J}_C}{\sigma I_0}$, we get:

$$L = \frac{-1}{I_0 \sigma} \vec{J}_C \cdot \vec{p}_H. \tag{5.25}$$

By comparing Eq. 5.25 with the extended Burger's equation 5.11 we see that the measured lead voltage is obtained as a scalar product of the heart vector and the lead vector $\frac{-1}{I_0 \sigma} \vec{J}_C$, which is independent of the location of $\vec{p}_H$. Consequently, if we were able to design a constant and known lead field, and under assumption of the volume source being homogeneous, we could obtain the heart vector $\vec{p}_H$ by using the procedure described in Sect. 5.3.3. In general, however, it is not practically possible to design a completely homogeneous lead field, because of the nature of the current distribution through a volume conductor, and because of the intrinsic inhomogeneity of real volume conductors.

An alternative, practical and applicable way of determining the heart dipole is the application of the Gabor-Nelson theorem, which, still under assumption of a homogeneous conductor, relates the heart dipole to the measurements of volume conductor surface potentials:

$$\vec{p}_H = \sigma \int_S \phi d\vec{S}, \tag{5.26}$$

where ϕ is the potential at the surface element $d\vec{S}$ and σ is the conductivity of the body surface S. The Gabor-Nelson theorem has been used to practically estimate the heart vector [18], but it can also be used to find the location of the heart vector [19].

Like image surfaces, the lead fields are also computed by using models of a volume conductor. Some examples of computed lead fields are found in [20], where a computer thorax model developed from CT-scans has been used. Another more recent model is from Horàček et al., who used a boundary-element model of a realistic three-dimensional human torso containing lungs and intracavity blood masses of different conductivities, to calculate lead vectors of 1239 heart vector locations, for 352 unipolar body-surface leads [17].

5.6 Lead System Design—Differential Lead Positioning

An additional consequence of the reciprocity theorem is that if we wanted to catch each source element $\vec{J^i}dV$ with the same weight, i.e., with the same sensitivity, we would need a homogeneous, i.e., constant lead field $\nabla\phi_0''$. This fact is the main design guideline behind all the vectorcardiography (VCG) lead systems. On the other hand, a lead system may be targeted to a specific part and/or side of the heart. This is accomplished by designing leads that have lead fields stronger (larger $|\nabla\phi_0''|$) in a particular segment of the heart.

Let us first consider the lead field for a point electrode. The potential field and its gradient for a monopole [13] are given by:

$$\phi_M = \frac{I_M}{4\pi\sigma}\frac{1}{r}, \quad \nabla\phi_M = -\frac{I_M}{4\pi\sigma}\frac{1}{r^2}\vec{a_r}, \tag{5.27}$$

where I_M is the monopole's source current strength, $\vec{r}$ is the radius vector for a point in space at which the field is evaluated, and $\vec{a_r}$ is the unit vector in the direction of $\vec{r}$. Since, according to Eq. 5.21, the lead field is equal to the gradient of the potential field caused by reciprocal current, $\nabla\phi_M$ is the lead field for a point electrode. From Eq. 5.27, it follows that $\nabla\phi_M$ decreases in magnitude with the square of the distance from the electrode. Consequently, this field will weight sources close to the electrode more heavily, by a square of the distance.

For a closely spaced electrode pair, also termed differential lead (DL), according to Eq. 5.21, the field will be the gradient of a dipole field. The potential field of a dipole $\vec{p}$ and its gradient [21] are given by:

$$\phi_D = \frac{\vec{a_r}\cdot\vec{p}}{4\pi\sigma}\frac{1}{r^2}, \quad \nabla\phi_D = -\frac{1}{4\pi\sigma}\frac{1}{r^3}[3(\vec{a_r}\cdot\vec{p})\vec{a_r} - \vec{p}], \tag{5.28}$$

which shows that a DL field weakens with the cube of the distance. Consequently, the source elements closer to the DL's electrodes' positions are weighted more strongly, by a factor of r^3. Therefore, DLs can be considered as very focused cardiac electrical activity detection devices. Moreover, DLs can be strategically placed so that their lead field obtains a particular property. Figure 5.4 illustrates the lead field of a DL.

It has been experimentally shown that DLs provide high quality ECG signals [22]. Most of the studies evaluating patch ECG monitors concentrate on arrhythmia detection. Studies done with a Philips experimental device featuring three DLs claim that the system provides high agreement with the EASI Holter monitor, in term of "evaluation of atrial activity, ventricular morphology, rhythm diagnosis" [23], as well as for "recognition of ventricular ectopic activity and ventricular fibrillation" [24]. An evaluation of Zio Patch [25] shows that the patch monitor detects more arrhythmic events than a conventional Holter monitor over the total wear time, but during 24-h it detected significantly less arrhythmic events than the Holter monitor. Clinical evaluation of the WPR Medical monitor shows better performance than the Holter monitor, but the authors conclude "that recorded ECG signals obtained from the wireless ECG system had an acceptable quality for arrhythmia diagnosis" [26]. An evaluation of the Imec's ECG patch shows, on ten subjects, that "the new ECG patch has the same performance as a medical gold standard Holter" for atrial fibrillation detection [27]. Also, an evaluation of the ePatch [28] shows that it can be useful for rhythm analysis.

Investigations of the applicability of DLs for specific purposes other than arrhythmia detection have been scarce so far. Investigations in [29] and [30] show that a DL can provide better sensitivity for detecting left ventricular hypertrophy than the Sokolow-Lyon criterion on the 12-lead ECG. Furthermore, the so-called CM5 lead—the lead between the manubrium and the V5 position—is commonly used as an additional lead to the 12-lead ECG during an exercise electrocardiographic test. A recent report shows that CM5 contributes to increased sensitivity of the exercise ECG to the coronary artery disease [31].

5.7 ECG Leads Synthesis from Three Measured Leads—General Considerations

Synthesis of leads is a process of transforming one lead system into another. Measurements are available for the lead system being transformed, whereas the leads for the newly produced system are not measured (or at least some of the leads are not measured directly). Even though such transformation can be obtained in various ways, and can even be nonlinear, it is worth to consider it first as a linear transformation of lead vectors. For obtaining a fixed, i.e. time independent, linear transformation between two lead systems, we will assume that the heart is a fixed-location dipole, the body is a linear system with time-invariant conductivity, and there is no noise in measurements.

Assume two lead systems $\mathbb{S}_1 = \{S_1^1, \ldots, S_1^{m_1}\}$ and $\mathbb{S}_2 = \{S_2^1, \ldots, S_2^{m_2}\}$ with m_1 and m_2 leads. Under the aforementioned assumptions, we may employ the Burger's equation for every lead in both systems and for an arbitrary point in time:

$$S_1 = \vec{S}_1 \cdot \vec{p}, \qquad S_2 = \vec{S}_2 \cdot \vec{p}, \tag{5.29}$$

where S_1 and S_2 are one-column matrices of lead values, $\vec{S}_1$ and $\vec{S}_2$ are the matrices with $\mathbb{S}_1$ and $\mathbb{S}_2$ systems' lead vectors in rows, and $\vec{p}$ is a fixed-location dipole describing the heart (column vector). The matrices $\vec{S}_1$ and $\vec{S}_2$ have dimensions $m_1 \times 3$ and $m_2 \times 3$, respectively. Since three independent leads are necessary for describing a fixed-location dipole (Sect. 5.3.3), we will assume that the rank of $\vec{S}_1$ and $\vec{S}_2$ is 3.

We are searching for a linear transformation X that transforms S_1 to S_2:

$$S_2 = X \cdot S_1. \tag{5.30}$$

By combining Eqs. 5.29 and 5.30, we obtain $\vec{S_2} \cdot \vec{p} = X \cdot \vec{S_1} \cdot \vec{p}$, which is true only if $\vec{S_2} = X \cdot \vec{S_1}$.

Under the above assumptions, just three independent leads are sufficient for uniquely obtaining the dipole $\vec{p}$. Therefore, only three independent leads from $\vec{S_1}$ are sufficient to obtain the transformation X. We will denote the matrix with three arbitrary, linearly independent leads from $\vec{S_1}$ as $\vec{S_1}^*$, so that we can write:

$$\vec{S_2} = X \cdot \vec{S_1}^*, \tag{5.31}$$

where $\vec{S_1}^*$ is a square 3×3 matrix with the full rank and, hence, the inverse matrix $(\vec{S_1}^*)^{-1}$ always exists. By multiplying Eq. 5.31 by $\vec{S_1}^{*^{-1}}$ from the right, we obtain:

$$X = \vec{S_2} \cdot (\vec{S_1}^*)^{-1}. \tag{5.32}$$

The equation tells how the linear transformation X between the lead systems $\mathbb{S}_1$ and $\mathbb{S}_2$ can be calculated directly from the lead vectors of both systems.

According to the discussion in Sect. 5.3.2, the lead vectors are obtained from a model of a human torso. By using such "generic" lead vectors for obtaining the transformation X, one is ignoring the individual characteristics of the volume conductor and the $\vec{p_H}$ locations, on which the lead vectors depend. For this reason, and since the assumptions we have made are in reality not completely satisfied, the transformed lead values $X \cdot S_1$ will in general deviate from the measured values, which can be expressed as:

$$S_2 = X \cdot S_1 + \vec{\varepsilon}, \tag{5.33}$$

where $\vec{\varepsilon}$ is a column vector of differences between the synthesized and the measured values for each lead.

The transformation X depends only on the lead vectors of the two lead systems. These lead vectors, and consequently the transformation X, are time-independent thanks to the assumption of a fixed heart vector and a constant conductivity. Still, if we are transforming between lead systems that have approximately homogeneous lead fields, i.e., similar lead vectors for different locations of the dipole, we can apply the transformation X without accepting that the heart dipole has a fixed location, i.e., by letting the dipole location to vary in time. This can be done because lead vectors in an approximately homogeneous lead field are similar in different locations.

If measurements from both lead systems $\mathbb{S}_1$ and $\mathbb{S}_2$ are a priori available for a person, it is obvious, from Eq. 5.33, that a personalized transformation X can be obtained with regression methods, even though there is no practical way of obtaining personalized lead vectors, as that would require a volume source and a volume conductor model to be constructed for each person. For that reason, researchers usually rely on regression to find a transformation between lead systems (more details in Sect. 5.8).

Regardless of the synthesis method, it is preferred that each lead picks up rich "information" about the cardiac electrical activity, preferably with complementary "information" from those parts of the heart where the other leads are weaker. By considering Eq. 5.24, this is accomplished with leads having lead fields strong in their particular parts of the heart, since it is not practically possible to construct lead fields of a constant strength. This also ensures an adequate signal-to-noise ratio for at least one lead at a certain instant of time.

An additional consideration is the orthogonality of the lead vectors. According to the Burger's equation, as the angle between $\vec{p}$ and $\vec{L}$ approaches $90°$, the measured voltage drops, which can cause a low signal-to-noise ratio for that lead. Therefore, we prefer orthogonal lead vectors, so that when $\vec{p}$ is nearly orthogonal to a certain lead, it has a large projection on at least one other lead vector.

5.7.1   Correctness of the Dipole Volume Source Model

The linear transformation X between two lead systems, derived in the previous section, relies on the dipole model and, hence, neglects all the information about the cardiac electrical activity not explained by the dipole. Consequently, X is only as good as the dipole is a correct approximation for an equivalent source.

The output of the VCG lead systems is the path of the heart's dipole tip during the heart cycle. Consequently, any evaluation of the diagnostic content of a VCG system is also an evaluation of the dipole volume source model. Even though VCG is almost extinct from today's electrocardiography, there are studies providing evidence that it contains practically the same diagnostic information as the standard 12-lead ECG [32].

The Becking-Burger technique [33] is a way of measuring the non-dipole components of cardiac electrical activity by evaluating the quality of a lead, preferably close to the heart, synthesized from three independent leads, preferably at some distance from the heart. Even though the Becking-Burger technique usually uses orthogonal lead systems, it is also possible to use an arbitrary set of three linearly independent reference leads. Any evaluation of the leads synthesized from a system of three linearly independent leads can be considered as applying the Becking-Burger technique to multiple leads, i.e. the leads of the synthesized system. One of the most comprehensive evaluations of a derived ECG system, namely the EASI lead system, was conducted by Horàček et al. [17, 34] on a population of 892 individuals, mostly patients with a previous myocardial infarction. The results of this study also support the correctness of the dipole hypothesis.

5.8   Overview of Methods for the Synthesis of the 12-Lead ECG

Both linear and nonlinear methods have been used to model relations between ECG leads for the purpose of lead synthesis [35, 36]. The linear regression has been the most often utilized method [35]. Among the nonlinear methods, artificial neural networks (NNs) have been mostly used [37].

Recent publications, besides traditional methods, like multiple linear regression [38], report also some novel approaches for ECG leads synthesis, like support vector regression [39], regression trees [40], and state-space models [41]. Some researchers apply linear transformation on independent [42] or principal components [43–45], or on derived characteristics in the wavelet domain [46], instead of transforming original signals. Even though the derived characteristics in general do not contain all the information from the original signal, such transformations can be justified by the fact that the independent and principal component analysis can be efficient noise-filtering methods.

The deterministic method described in Sect. 5.7 was also sometimes used. This method takes lead vectors from an image surface and calculates the transformation matrix according to Eq. 5.32. Cao et al. used the deterministic approach to synthesize the 12-lead ECG from three DLs [47]. Rarely used is also the search method. Its concept is to form different transformation matrices X by incrementing elements in X by a predefined value. Among all the transformations X obtained in this way, the best X is the one that synthesizes the 12-lead ECG that is, in terms of the employed metrics, most similar to the target ECG. The metrics for comparing ECGs are presented in the next section.

5.9 Synthesis Evaluation

The quality of the synthesized 12-lead ECG is evaluated by comparing it to the target 12-lead ECGs obtained in the standard way. The most commonly used metrics for automatic evaluation are the root-mean-square distance (RMSD) and the correlation coefficient (CC). In parallel with these methods, it is often useful to engage an expert, i.e. a cardiologist, to examine independently the target and the synthesized ECGs. The synthesis is considered to be successful if both ECGs lead the cardiologist to the same conclusions.

5.10 Synthesis Personalization

The synthesis of the 12-lead ECG can be universal or adjusted to each person. Although, in general, both the transformation parameters and the electrode positions can be personalized, almost all existing derived 12-lead ECG systems employ universal electrode positions. An exception are the patch ECG body sensors that can be placed in an arbitrary position on the body surface, meaning that their positions can be personalized [48]. The transformations, on the other hand, are universal or personalized. The transformation matrix is generally calculated from the lead vectors (see Sect. 5.7). Any personalization of the transformation matrix can, therefore, be considered as an employment of personalized lead vectors.

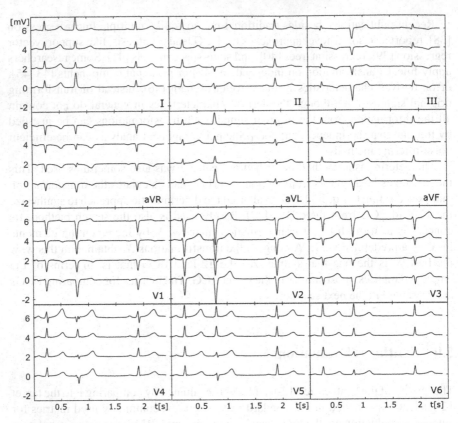

Fig. 5.5 Target 12-lead ECG (the bottom curve in each panel) and three synthesized 12-lead ECGs (the curves moved up by 2, 4 and 6 mV) drawn in this bottom-up order: (*I*) personalized DL positions and personalized transformation, (*II*) universal DL positions and personalized transformation, (*III*) universal DL positions and universal transformation. The second beat is an extrasystole

Since it is not practically possible to obtain personalized lead vectors (Sect. 5.7), the personalized synthesis requires simultaneous measurement of the 12-lead ECG and the leads used for the synthesis, which have to be obtained for each person before the transformation can be calculated with, e.g., linear regression or NNs. The universal synthesis, on the other hand, can be obtained by using an image space, or with NNs or linear regression, whose inputs are obtained by juxtaposing measurements from different individuals [35].

There are two additional methods for the universal synthesis. One forms the universal transformation coefficients as the mean of the transformation coefficients obtained for each person. The other method is a modification of the search method: instead of assuming the best combination of parameters to be the one that produces the best synthesized ECG for a particular person, the selected transformation coefficients are those that result in the best synthesis, on average, over all considered measurements.

The advantage of a universal synthesis is that, once calculated, the transformation parameters can be applied to every person without a need for new measurements. The disadvantage is that a universal synthesis generally gives results that are inferior to those obtained by a personalized approach, because the universal transformation parameters are not adjusted to the anatomical uniqueness of each person.

As for the synthesis from DLs, there have been a few investigations showing that a reliable 12-lead ECG can be synthesized from them, with the personalized approach providing the best results [47–50]. Figure 5.5 shows a 12-lead ECG obtained from a cardiac patient (the bottom curve in each panel). The synthesized 12-lead ECGs are presented with the upper three curves. They have been obtained from three DLs, but with different approaches (in the bottom-up order): (I) personalized DL positions and personalized transformation, (II) universal DL positions and personalized transformation, and (III) universal positions and universal transformation. All ECG curves are visually alike, but a detailed analysis confirms that the first approach provides an ECG most similar to the target ECG.

The second beat of the target ECG from Fig. 5.5 is an extrasystole, which is synthesized appropriately in most of the leads, except in the leads II, aVR, aVL and V5. Extrasystoles are harder to synthesize because they can have a different electrical origin than the normal beats, which implies different heart vector positions. For this reason, extrasystoles can be considered as a rigorous input to a synthesis evaluation. Both DL positions and transformations could be tailored to extrasistolic events, and this is an interesting future research topic.

The universal DL positions used in the synthesis of the two upper ECG curves from Fig. 5.5 are shown in Fig. 5.6, marked by A, B, and C. They were found by using an algorithm published in [49]. The same algorithm was used to obtain the best personalized DL positions. The algorithm uses all the unipolar leads defined by the electrodes marked in Fig. 5.6 with black circles, to find three DLs that provide

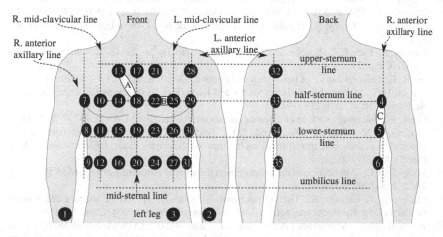

Fig. 5.6 35-channel ECG electrode positioning. The leads marked by *A*, *B*, and *C* are calculated as the best DLs for the 12-lead ECG synthesis

the best synthesis results. To find the universal DL positions marked in Fig. 5.6, the algorithm accepts juxtaposed ECG measurements from a number of patients and healthy persons, whereas for the personalized synthesis, the algorithm is fed with measurements from a single person. The best combination of three DLs provided by the algorithm is the one that produces synthesized 12-lead ECG with the biggest CC (see Sect. 5.9) to the target 12-lead ECG. For the synthesis from each triplet of DLs, linear regression was used.

References

1. Rush, S., Abildskov, J.A., McFee, R.: Resistivity of body tissues at low frequencies. Circ. Res. **12**, 40–50 (1963)
2. Schwan, H.P., Kay, C.F.: The conductivity of living tissues. Ann. N. Y. Acad. Sci. **65**(6), 1007–1013 (1957)
3. Plonsey, R., Heppner, D.B.: Considerations of quasi-stationarity in electrophysiological systems. Bull. Math. Biophy. **29**(4), 657–664 (1967)
4. Frank, E.: Spread of current in volume conductors of finite extent. Ann. N. Y. Acad. Sci. **65**(6), 980–1002 (1957)
5. Malmivuo, J., Plosney, R.: Forward and inverse problem. In: Bioelectromagnetism. Oxford University Press (1995) (Chap. 7.5)
6. Geselowitz, D.: On bioelectric potentials in an inhomogeneous volume conductor. Biophys. J. **7**(1), 1–11 (1967)
7. Geselowitz, D.B.: Dipole theory in electrocardiography. Am. J. Cardiol. **14**(3), 301–306 (1964)
8. Einthoven, W.: The different forms of the human electrocardiogram and their signification. Lancet **179**(4622), 853–861 (1912) (originally published as Volume 1, Issue 4622)
9. Einthoven, W., Fahr, G., Waart, A.: Über die richtung und die manifeste grösse der potentialschwankungen im menschlichen herzen und über den einfluss der herzlage auf die form des elektrokardiogramms. Pflüger's Archiv für die gesamte Physiologie des Menschen und der Tiere **150**(6), 275–315 (1913)
10. Burger, H.C., Milaan, J.B.V.: Heart-vector and leads. Br. Heart J. **8**(3), 157–161 (1946)
11. Burger, H.C., Milaan, J.B.V.: Heart-vector and leads. Part ii. Br. Heart J. **9**(3), 154–160 (1947)
12. Malmivuo, J., Plosney, R.: Dipole. In: Bioelectromagnetism. Oxford University Press (1995) (Chap. 8.2)
13. Plonsey, R., Barr, R.C.: Sources and fields. In: Bioelectricity, pp. 23–43, 3rd edn. Springer, US (2007) (Chap. 2)
14. Frank, E.: General theory of heart-vector projection. Circ. Res. **2**(3), 258–270 (1954)
15. Burger, H.C., Milaan, J.B.V.: Heart-vector and leads. Part III (Geometrical Representation). Br. Heart J. **10**(4), 229–233 (1948)
16. Frank, E.: The image surface of a homogeneous torso. Am. Heart J. **47**(5), 757–768 (1954)
17. Horácek, B.M., Warren, J.W., Feild, D.Q., Feldman, C.L.: Statistical and deterministic approaches to designing transformations of electrocardiographic leads. J. Electrocardiol. **35**(4, Part B), 41–52 (2002)
18. Voukydis, P.C.: Application of the gabor-nelson theory in electrocardiography. Med. Biol. Eng. **10**(2), 223–229 (1972)
19. Malmivuo, J., Plosney, R.: Theoretical methods for analyzing volume sources and volume conductors. In: Bioelectromagnetism. Oxford University Press (1995) (Chap. 11)
20. Hyttinen, J.A.K., Malmivuo, J.A., Walker, S.J.: Lead field of ECG leads calculated by a computer thorax model-an application of reciprocity. In: Proceedings of Computers in Cardiology, pp. 241–244 (1993)

21. Griffiths, D.J.: The electric field of a dipole. In: Introduction to Electrodynamics, pp. 153–155, 3rd edn. Prentice Hall (1999) (Chap. 3.4.4)

22. Puurtinen, M., Viik, J., Hyttinen, J.: Best electrode locations for a small bipolar ECG device: signal strength analysis of clinical data. Ann. Biomed. Eng. **37**(2), 331–336 (2009)

23. Janata, A., Lemmert, M.E., Russell, J.K., Gehman, S., Fleischhackl, R., Robak, O., Pernicka, E., Sterz, F., Gorgels, A.P.: Quality of ECG monitoring with a miniature ECG recorder. Pacing Clin. Electrophysiol. **31**(6), 676–684 (2008)

24. Lemmert, M.E., Janata, A., Erkens, P., Russell, J.K., Gehman, S., Nammi, K., Crijns, H.J., Sterz, F., Gorgels, A.P.: Detection of ventricular ectopy by a novel miniature electrocardiogram recorder. J. Electrocardiol. **44**(2), 222–228 (2011)

25. Barrett, P.M., Komatireddy, R., Haaser, S., Topol, S., Sheard, J., Encinas, J., Fought, A.J., Topol, E.J.: Comparison of 24-hour Holter monitoring with 14-day Novel adhesive patch electrocardiographic monitoring. Am. J. Med. **127**(1), 95.e11–95.e17 (2014)

26. Fensli, R., Gundersen, T., Snaprud, T., Hejlesen, O.: Clinical evaluation of a wireless ECG sensor system for arrhythmia diagnostic purposes. Med. Eng. Phys. **35**(6), 697–703 (2013)

27. Torfs, T., Smeets, C.J., Geng, D., Berset, T., der Auwera, J.V., Vandervoort, P., Grieten, L.: Clinical validation of a low-power and wearable ECG patch for long term full-disclosure monitoring. J. Electrocardiol. **47**(6), 881–889 (2014)

28. Saadi, D., Fauerskov, I., Osmanagic, A., Sheta, H., Sorensen, H., Egstrup, K., Hoppe, K.: Heart rhythm analysis using ECG recorded with a novel sternum based patch technology: a pilot study. In: Proceedings of the International Congress on Cardiovascular Technologies (CARDIOTECHNIX), pp. 15–21 (2013)

29. Väisänen, J., Puurtinen, M., Hyttinen, J., Viik, J.: Short Distance bipolar electrocardiographic leads in diagnosis of left ventricular hypertrophy. Comput. Cardiol. **37**, 293–296 (2010)

30. Puurtinen, M., Väisänen, J., Viik, J., Hyttinen, J.: New precordial bipolar electrocardiographic leads for detecting left ventricular hypertrophy. J. Electrocardiol. **43**(6), 654–659 (2010)

31. Puurtinen, M., Nieminen, T., Kähönen, M., Lehtimäki, T., Lehtinen, R., Nikus, K., Hyttinen, J., Viik, J.: Value of leads V4R and CM5 in the detection of coronary artery disease during exercise electrocardiographic test. Clin. Physiol. Funct. Imaging **30**(4), 308–312 (2010)

32. Willems, J.L., Lesaffre, E., Pardaens, J.: Comparison of the classification ability of the electrocardiogram and vectorcardiogram. Am. J. Cardiol. **59**(1), 119–124 (1987)

33. Burger, H.C.: Lead vector projections. I., Ann. N. Y. Acad. Sci. **65**(6), 1076–1087 (1957)

34. Horáček, B.M., Warren, J.W., Stóvícek, P., Feldman, C.L.: Diagnostic accuracy of derived versus standard 12-lead electrocardiograms. J. Electrocardiol. **33**(Supplement 1), 155–160 (2000)

35. Tomašić, I., Trobec, R.: Electrocardiographic systems with reduced numbers of leads – Synthesis of the 12-lead ECG. IEEE Rev. Biomed. Eng. **7**, 126–142 (2014)

36. Vozda, M., Cerny, M.: Methods for derivation of orthogonal leads from 12-lead electrocardiogram: a review. Biomed. Signal Process. Control **19**, 23–34 (2015)

37. Atoui, H., Fayn, J., Rubel, P.: A novel neural-network model for deriving standard 12-lead ECGs from serial three-lead ECGs: application to self-care. IEEE Trans. Inform. Technol. Biomed. **14**(3), 883–890 (2010)

38. Figueiredo, C.P., Mendes, P.M.: Towards wearable and continuous 12-lead electrocardiogram monitoring: Synthesis of the 12-lead electrocardiogram using 3 wireless single-lead sensors. In: Proceedings of the International Conference on Biomedical Electronics and Devices (BIODEVICES), pp. 329–332 (2012)

39. Yodjaiphet, A., Theera-Umpon, N., Auephanwiriyakul, S.: Electrocardiogram reconstruction using support vector regression. In: Proceedings of the IEEE International Symposium on Signal Processing and Information Technology (ISSPIT), pp. 000269–000273 (2012)

40. Tomasic, I., Trobec, R., Lindén, M.: Can the regression trees be used to model relation between ECG leads? In: Internet of Things. IoT Infrastructures: Second International Summit, pp. 467–472. Springer International Publishing (2016)

41. Lee, J., Kim, M., Kim, J.: Reconstruction of precordial lead electrocardiogram from limb leads using the state-space model. IEEE J. Biomed. Health Informat. **20**(3), 818–828 (2016)

42. Tsouri, G.R., Ostertag, M.H.: Patient-specific 12-lead ECG reconstruction from sparse electrodes using independent component analysis. IEEE J. Biomed. Health Informat. **18**(2), 476–482 (2014)
43. Tomašić, I., Skala, K., Trobec, R.: Principal component analysis and visualization in optimization and personalization of lead's set for generation of standard 12-leads ECG. In: Proceedings of the 31th International Convention on Information and Communication Technology, Electronics and Microelectronics, pp. 307–313 (2008)
44. Mann, S., Orglmeister, R.: PCA-based ECG lead reconstruction. Biomedizinische Technik. Biomed. Eng. **58**(Supp. 1), 24–25 (2013)
45. Dawson, D., Yang, H., Malshe, M., Bukkapatnam, S.T.S., Benjamin, B., Komanduri, R.: Linear affine transformations between 3-lead (Frank XYZ leads) vectorcardiogram and 12-lead electrocardiogram signals. J. Electrocardiol. **42**(6), 622–630 (2009)
46. Nallikuzhy, J.J., Dandapat, S.: Enhancement of the spatial resolution of ECG using multi-scale Linear Regression. In: Proceedings of the 21st National Conference on Communications (NCC), pp. 1–6 (2015)
47. Cao, H., Li, H., Stocco, L., Leung, V.C.M.: Wireless three-pad ECG system: challenges, design, and evaluations. J. Commun. Netw. **13**(2), 113–124 (2011)
48. Trobec, R., Tomašić, I.: Synthesis of the 12-lead electrocardiogram from differential leads. IEEE Trans. Inf. Technol. Biomed. **15**(4), 615–621 (2011)
49. Tomašić, I., Frljak, S., Trobec, R.: Estimating the universal positions of wireless body electrodes for measuring cardiac electrical activity. IEEE Trans. Inf. Technol. Biomed. **60**(12), 3368–3374 (2013)
50. Hansen, I.H., Hoppe, K., Gjerde, A., Kanters, J.K., Sorensen, H.B.D.: Comparing twelve-lead electrocardiography with close-to-heart patch based electrocardiography. In: Proceedings of the 37th Annual International Conference of the IEEE Engineering in Medicine and Biology Society (EMBC), pp. 330–333 (2015)

Chapter 6
Commercial ECG Systems

Abstract Besides the standard 12-lead ECG and the Holter monitor, today the market offers a wide range of modern ECG devices and services supported by the latest developments in ICT. This chapter is devoted to the current state-of-the-art from the area of ECG with a reduced number of leads. We focus on ECG wireless body sensors, differentiating between those that measure only heart rate and are used just for entertainment or during sport activities, and those that actually measure and analyze the ECG signal, with all its waveforms. The latter are elaborated in more detail, particularly our differential ECG sensor and its commercial version Savvy, for which we provide also a comprehensive comparison to other state-of-the-art sensors in that field. It is, however, inevitable that the state-of-the art will change in the future. The constant progress in ICT will always drive the development of new and improved ECG devices.

6.1 Advances in ECG Monitoring Supported by ICT

The development of ICT has reached a level where its usefulness can be applied for healthcare needs towards Telemedicine and Telecare [1–4], which represent a promising alternative for today's traditional hospital admission. This basic premise is included in all strategic plans of the EU and the rest of the world [5–7]. Studies have clearly concluded that regular acquisition of clinical and physiological data of high-risk patients through wireless technologies provides a good model for clinical decision-making, determining better quality of life and reducing mortality and hospitalizations [8]. Several technological solutions for mHealth, based on mobile network infrastructure with smartphones and Internet connection, have been proposed [1]. It is evident that such ICT solutions have a great potential for the optimization of the economic aspects of health treatment; however, no solution is widely accepted.

6.1.1 ECG Services in Sports and Entertainment

Numerous ECG sensors and associated mHealth services are already available, from those used just for entertainment and in sports, to more professional ones, intended

© The Author(s) 2018
R. Trobec et al., *Body Sensors and Electrocardiography*, SpringerBriefs
in Applied Sciences and Technology, DOI 10.1007/978-3-319-59340-1_6

101

for medical use. Monitoring the heart in sports is done mostly for determining only the heart rate. Therefore, the detection of the QRS complex in the ECG signal is sufficient and the quality of the recordings is less important. Consequently, for use in sports, simpler ways of signal acquisition are being utilized, for example, a belt with conducting parts, which is attached around the chest. Chest belt systems with wireless transmission are used in sports and for medical monitoring, where in the latter case, at least a bipolar leads ECG signal with a reasonable sampling accuracy is provided. An example is the CorBELT event recorder from Corescience GmbH & Co. KG, Germany.[1]

In the field of health monitoring applications on smartphones, all applications are intended for individuals for approximate and unreliable assessments, for example, of the heart rhythm. The applications are based on optical evaluation of the light reflected from the tissue, as detected by the camera device. The pulsating blood flow modulates the light, which allows for the heart rate to be determined. Examples of such applications are the Instant Heart Rate app, developed by Azumio, avaliable for iOS[2] and Android,[3] or the Heart Rate app from Plus Sports, available for iOS.[4] Most of the more professional applications on smartphones are bundled with the purchase of a sensor and are adapted for integration into the health monitoring system, so that the purchase of these services is possible only as a package. The current most widely used mobile sensor—the Holter, contains in the package also a web application. The communication protocol between the sensor and the application is not open, preventing the development of competitive applications. Nevertheless, there are several freely accessible applications available specifically for medical practitioners and intended to assist them in ECG measurement and prognosis. Among them is also the VisECG application that was developed in collaboration between the Clinical Center Ljubljana and the Department of Communication Systems at the Jožef Stefan Institute [9, 10].

6.1.2 Medical ECG Devices

In the areas of professional ECG devices and services intended for medical use, the advances in ICT have enabled more mobile ECG services, compared to the Holter monitor. One of the new solutions is the CardioSecur system from Personal MedSystems GmbH, Germany[5] (Fig. 6.1a). It is multi-lead and still uses wires, but offers advanced online ECG diagnostic. The device is CE marked as a class IIa medical product. It consists of four electrodes that must be positioned on specified

---

[1]https://www.corscience.com/.

[2]https://itunes.apple.com/us/app/instant-heart-rate-heart-rate/id409625068?mt=8.

[3]https://play.google.com/store/apps/details?id=si.modula.android.instantheartrate&hl=en.

[4]https://itunes.apple.com/us/app/heart-rate-monitor-measure/id795738018?mt=8.

[5]https://www.cardiosecur.com.

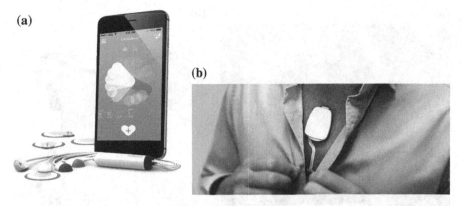

Fig. 6.1 **a** CardioSecur system from Personal MedSystems GmbH. Picture taken from the company's web site https://www.cardiosecur.com (accessed on Jan 27, 2017). **b** ePatch® from DELTA Danish Electronics, Light & Acoustics. Picture taken from the company's web site http://epatch. madebydelta.com (accessed on Jan 27, 2017)

locations on the body and then connected via the CardioSecur ACTIVE mobile ECG cable to a smartphone. The device is accompanied by a CardioSecur ACTIVE application that allows the user to record a reference ECG. When symptoms occur or the user wants to perform a checkup of the heart, a control ECG is recorded and compared to the reference ECG. The application then gives recommendations on how to act: Neutral—no abnormalities compared to the reference ECG, Yellow—plan a visit to the doctor, and Red—see a doctor immediately. The ECG reading and report are immediately available within the application, on the user's online account, or they can also be shared with a physician. There is also a PRO version of CardioSecur, intended for physicians[6] with the option of an automatic diagnosis.

Other solutions offer multi-lead readings acquired by a single patch, like the ePatch®, originally developed by DELTA Danish Electronics, Light & Acoustics, now a part of BioTelemetry Inc., Denmark[7] (Fig. 6.1b). The ePatch® is CE marked and FDA cleared, and adheres to regulatory Holter standards. It is a small single multi-lead patch, without cables, weighs only 16 g and offers a more mobile Holter option. It consists of a sensor and a patch. The ePatch® sensor is first inserted into the patch. The patch is then adhered to the skin and the ePatch® starts recording. It continuously records and stores 1–3 channels ECG for up to 72 h. An event marker function is available via a double tap on the sensor. The readings are recorded in the internal storage of the sensor. After recording, the data is read out on a PC via USB interface cable and analyzed using a dedicated web services or software installed on the PC. However, these multi-lead ECG solutions still do not offer online

---

[6]http://mobile-ecg.com.

[7]http://epatch.madebydelta.com.

(a)   (b)

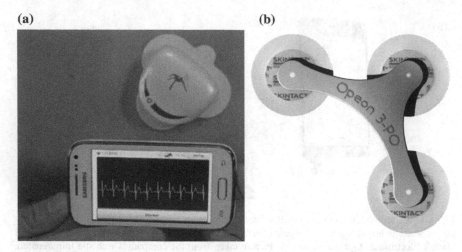

Fig. 6.2 **a** Spyder sensor from WEB Biotechnology Pte Ltd. Picture taken from the company's web site http://www.web-biotech.com (accessed on Jan 27, 2017). **b** Cortrium C3 from Cortrium. Picture taken from the company's web site http://cortrium.com (accessed on Jan 27, 2017)

wireless transmission of data. Two solutions that do provide such option are the Spyder BT sensor from WEB Biotechnology Pte Ltd, Singapore[8] (Fig. 6.2a) and Cortrium C3 from Cortrium, Denmark[9] (Fig. 6.2b), but they are still not certified as medical devices.

The recent trend in ECG device development is towards wireless leadless differential ECG sensors. An example is the commercial system for heart rate monitoring—LifeTouch Patient Surveillance System from Isansys Lifecare, Great Britain, illustrated in Fig. 6.3. It is a class IIa CE marked medical device. The LifeTouch sensor is attached to the patient's chest using standard and replaceable ECG electrodes, and activated with a pull tab. The body sensor measures heart rate with a resolution of milliseconds and respiratory rate (derived from the ECG), and has a data connection, over a near-installed special router, to a server that provides support services. The connection to the server is via a mobile terminal with Bluetooth Smart technology. The LifeTouch sensor was promoted as the "World's First Cloud-Ready Medical Device". The sensor measures just the heart rate, which allows an assessment of the heart rate variability. However, it does not measure the ECG with an adequate sampling rate needed for detailed analysis. The ECG visualization function is only for the purpose of setup and verification. Thus, the area of mobile ECG monitoring remains open for further improvement. In the rest of the chapter, we focus on more advanced differential leadless ECG sensors.

---

[8]http://www.web-biotech.com.
[9]http://cortrium.com.

Fig. 6.3 ECG body sensor
from Isansys Lifecare.
Picture taken from the
company's web site http://
www.isansys.com (accessed
on Dec 8, 2016)

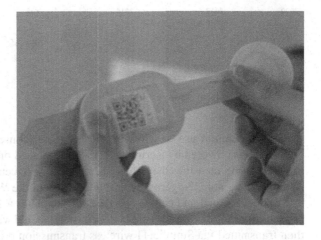

6.2 Differential ECG Wireless Body Sensors

The idea that we have been working on for several years is to design a body gadget
based on a minimal number of body sensors with different functions, preferably all
combined in a single one, which will provide synchronized vital bio-signs of the
monitored user [11]. We have been in search for a system solution with the potential to become available for everybody at a cost similar to that of devices for blood
pressure monitoring at home, currently widespread among hypertensive patients.
The multichannel ECG with 64 electrodes on the surface of the body inspired our
solution. We recognized that a significant amount of information about heart activity could be measured just through the electric potential between two neighboring
multichannel electrodes. Such an approach enables non-invasive measurement with a
single-channel of bipolar ECG without wires. More details about how the implementation of wearable ECG sensors is connected to the multichannel ECG is provided in
Chap. 2. Thus, our solution is situated between the Holter monitor and the implantable
loop recorder (ILR) with the possibility of immediate access to the measured data.
With appropriate placement of the device on the chest, good visibility of all electrocardiographic waves (P, QRS and T) can be achieved, allowing for quality ECG
recording sufficient for medical analysis. In contrast, implanted ECG recorders often
record P waves that are poorly visible or not visible at all. Compared to the Holter
monitor, our solution is open source, wireless, and low-cost. Moreover, it has already
been used for research purposes.

The device in its current design is a result of almost 7 years of research, development, testing and upgrades. In Fig. 6.4, the evolution of the sensor design is presented.
As an initial design, we prototyped a differential wireless body sensor (WBS) for
measuring ECG and EEG [12]. An example of the prototype is shown in Fig. 6.4,
year 2009. The WBS consists of two self-adhesive electrodes (which need to be
positioned at a distance of 5 cm when performing measurements), a signal amplifier, a micro-controller and a low-power 2.4 GHz radio (Texas Instruments CC2500).

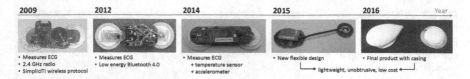

Fig. 6.4 Wireless body sensor evolution

It enables minimal use of wires on the body and consequently maximal wearing comfort. It is powered by a coin battery. When placed on the body surface near the heart, the WBS measures the potential difference between the electrodes and records a raw ECG signal. Triggered by an internal clock, the WBS performs sampling of the analogue signal and conversion of each sample to a 10-bit digital signal. Seven consecutive samples are collected into a buffer, labeled with a source time stamp and then transmitted via SimpliciTI wireless transmission protocol.[10]

The initial design was later upgraded to support the newest version of the Bluetooth technology—Bluetooth low energy (BLE)—for transmission of measured data from the WBS. Thereby we enabled direct communication between the WBS and smartphones and devices with incorporated low energy Bluetooth. An example of the prototype is shown in Fig. 6.4, year 2012. The Bluetooth low energy protocol is a low-cost wireless solution designed to meet special requirements for long-term operation in devices with limited energy capacity (e.g. with a coin-cell battery). Its ultra-low peak, average and idle mode power consumption and enhanced working range enable the WBS to operate on a single coin-cell battery for several days while transmitting a live stream of raw ECG data [13]. The maximal bit-rate of the data payload is 1 Mb/s, which is sufficient also for high-resolution short-term measurements.

Our next concern was to improve data collection. Starting with the version presented in Fig. 6.4, year 2014, the WBS incorporates more sensors, like a temperature sensor and an accelerometer, making it a multi-functional wireless body sensor (MWBS). Furthermore, other relevant data can be extracted from the raw ECG signal using additional signal processing. First, the WBS provides an alternative that resolves the standard 12-lead ECG devices imperfections. The measurements from three WBSs can form a lead system that can potentially be used for the reconstruction of the 12-lead ECG [14, 15]. Next, we have confirmed that the WBS measurements can be also used for monitoring the respiration frequency and for rough classification of the breathing types by using ECG-derived respiration (EDR) techniques [16]. EDR techniques are based on the observation that the positions of the ECG electrodes on the chest surface move relative to the heart.

The latest version of the sensor has a more flexible lightweight design that allows for unobtrusive long-term mobile health monitoring (Fig. 6.4, year 2015). The electrodes are connected with a small wire at a distance of 8 cm (bipolar lead) [11]. This sensor is in the center of a system for mobile monitoring of vital physiological para-

---

[10]http://www.ti.com/simpliciti.

meters and the environmental context [17], registered as a technology innovation at the Jožef Stefan Institute since 2015. Such design of the sensor allows for a low-cost implementation with an appropriate casing (Fig. 6.4, year 2016). The know-how of our technological invention was successfully transferred to a medical company and the required medical certificates: MDD 93/42/EEC, EN 60601 and EN ISO 14971, have been obtained. A commercial version of the medically certified ECG sensor[11] is available on the market since 2016.

6.2.1 Savvy Sensor

The medical device is a Personal device for CARDiac activity (PCARD)—trademarked Savvy ECG. It represents a set of basic equipment and accessories. The basic equipment includes: a body gadget—Savvy sensor with battery charger (Fig. 6.5), a mobile application (MobECG), and stand-alone software for visualization and basic analysis of the measured ECG (VisECG) on a safe storage server. Accessories that are needed for proper operation of the medical device are: medically certified self-adhesive electrodes, a personal digital assistant (PDA), like a smartphone or a tablet, and either a safe storage server or Cloud platform. The core of the system is the Savvy sensor—a small and light body gadget fixed to the skin of the user by two standard self-adhesive electrodes. Only two electrical connectors are required on the Savvy sensor. These two connecting points are used (i) to connect the electrodes and perform measurements in measuring mode, and (ii) to plug the sensor on the battery charger in charging mode. The battery charger is implemented as a charging dock and is designed in a way that hinders short circuits between the AC/DC outputs, their contact with the user's skin, and reverse connection of the Savvy sensor. The sensor is covered with a waterproof and biocompatible plastic housing. The flexible mechanical construction of the Savvy sensor housing and the flexible connection to the electrodes enable adaptation of the distance between the two electrodes, which prevents an unexpected disconnection of the Savvy sensor during user's movements. For optimal power consumption, the ECG is recorded with a moderate resolution of 125 samples per second, but the sampling rate can be increased. With a single charge of the built-in battery, the Savvy sensor can run continuously up to 10 days or up to 20 days in stand-by mode. More details about measurements with the sensor are provided in Chap. 2.

 The mobile application is installed on the PDA and its main functionalities include: establishing communication between the Savvy sensor and the PDA, visualization of the ongoing measurement, storing the measured data on the PDA storage, interaction with the user, and transferring the measurements to a secure storage server or Cloud platform. More details about the mobile application are provided in Chap. 3. A special added value of the system is the visualization program used to review and analyze the measurements after they are finished. The MobECG program has an option to

---

[11] http://savvy.si/.

(a)   (b)

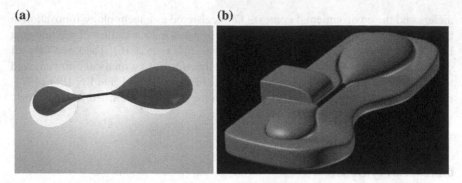

Fig. 6.5 Savvy sensor **a** The wearable body sensor in biocompatible housing with two self-adhesive electrodes attached. **b** The body sensor during charging, placed in the charging dock

generate a summary ECG report of a measurement around a user's marked event. The ECG report can be shared with a trusted caregiver or a medical expert. After the measurements have been stored on a computer, the VisECG program can provide a more detailed ECG report of all measurements. For each ECG measurement in the report, the mean heart rate per minute is plotted with a line and all instantaneous heart rates are displayed as dots. The events which were marked during the measurement, e.g., when some activity was initiated or when some inconvenience has been felt, are marked on the graphs together with a minute interval of the ECG signal around the marked event. The ECG report is not intended for diagnostic purposes, but as a preliminary indication for medical doctors if some threatening arrhythmias have been present during a long-term measurement, which can last from a few days to a month. An example of a VisECG report is shown in Fig. 6.6.

6.2.2 Comparison of the Savvy Sensor with Related ECG Sensors

A literature search was made to find devices that are equivalent to the Savvy sensor, regarding safety and performance, and declared as CE-marked and/or FDA-approved leadless noninvasive (patch) ECG devices. For evaluation with the Savvy ECG system, the data for comparison with equivalent devices is taken from [18]. In Table 6.1, the Savvy sensor is compared to two equivalent devices, ZIO® XT and SEEQ™, shown in Fig. 6.7.

The main difference between the Savvy ECG system and the other two devices is that the Savvy sensor has a rechargeable battery and is reusable, while the other two are not. If the user accepts the Savvy sensor in tandem with his/her smartphone as a personal ECG sensor, the whole Savvy system becomes a long-term ECG monitoring system. The ZIO® XT patch is applied on the body once for up to 14 days and then

Fig. 6.6 VisECG report example

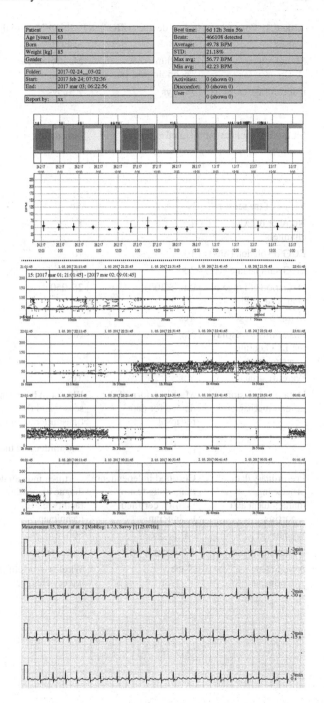

Table 6.1 Comparison of two devices (ZIO® XT, SEEQ™) with the Savvy sensor

Sensor	ZIO® XT	SEEQ™	Savvy
Manufacturer	iRhythm Technologies, Inc.	Medtronic, Inc.	Saving d.o.o.
Data storage capacity	14 days	7.5 days	More than 30 days (limited by the PDA capacity)
Method of application	Timed adhesive	Timed adhesive	Standard adhesive ECG electrodes for 3 days. Successive application after recharging the sensor
Reuse of the sensor	No	No	Yes
Number of ECG channels	1	1	1
ECG resolution (bits)	10	16	10
ECG sample rate (Hz)	200	200	125
Detection of range of heart rate (BPM)	0 to >300	25–250	20–250
Symptom trigger	Yes	Yes	Yes
Possibility to display the ECG during measurement	No	No	Yes
Water resistant	Yes	Yes	Yes
Data transmission or upload mechanism	Mail-in return of the device for data retrieval	Bluetooth between the sensor and the transmitter, cellular between the transmitter and the server	Bluetooth between the sensor and the PDA, WiFi between the PDA and the server
Preliminary data processing, management and reporting	Certified independent diagnostic testing facility, certified technician	Certified independent diagnostic testing facility, certified technician	Computer assisted viewing and analysis tool (VisECG)
Weight (g)	34	50	21
Dimensions (mm)	123 × 53 × 10.7	160 × 60 × 15	130 × 35 × 14
Associated components	None	Wireless transmitter, battery charger	Smartphone or tablet, battery charger, standard ECG electrodes

Fig. 6.7 **a** ZIO® XT Patch by iRhythm Technologies, Inc. Picture taken from the company's web site http://www.irhythmtech.com (accessed on Dec 8, 2016). **b** SEEQ™ sensor by Medtronic, Inc. Picture taken from the company's web site http://www.medtronicdiagnostics.com (accessed on Dec 8, 2016)

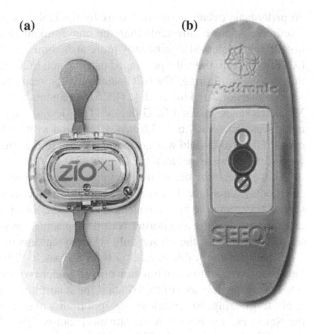

(a) (b)

returned by post to the company's ZIO ECG Utilization Service for study with no output during measurement time. On the other hand, the SEEQ™ system (two-piece design) has a possibility to transmit data in real time to the company's data network through a special transmitter device (cellular data transmission, zLink®), but the response time again depends on the time required for data processing by the company's Monitoring Center. The SEEQ™ sensor is applied to the body once, for a period of up to 7.5 days, with the possibility of deploying multiple different units for up to 30 days (up to 3 additional sensor units). The Savvy ECG system also has a two-piece design, where the first piece is the Savvy sensor on the body and the second piece is user's own smartphone (or tablet) in the vicinity. The smartphone/tablet is used to store and display the ECG and also as an input device through which the user can mark events in the recording. The ZIO® XT and SEEQ™ systems have for event marking only a push button on the sensor itself. Although the standard sampling frequency of the Savvy sensor is lower (125 Hz) than that of the other two systems (200 Hz), it is sufficient for post processing of the recordings. Studies have confirmed that the sampling frequency of 125 Hz is sufficient for heart rate variability detection if signal interpolation is applied [19]. Many of the Holter ECG systems also have sampling frequency of 125 Hz. The weight of the Savvy body sensor is the lowest from all the three compared systems.

Performance Evaluation

In a clinical research study, Barret et al. [20] compared 14-day single-channel adhesive ECG patch monitoring with conventional 24-h Holter monitoring on 146 patients for detection of arrhythmia events. The results showed that the patch monitor detected

96 arrhythmia events compared to 61 by the Holter monitor. Patients found patch monitoring more comfortable than the conventional Holter. Although the conventional Holter detected significantly more arrhythmias in the first 24-h than the patch ECG in the same time, the prolonged use of patch ECG overcompensated this in further days of monitoring. The ECG patch monitor wear time was in average 11.1 days.

In a study of Turakhia et al. [21], 26751 patients were monitored with the ZIO® XT patch single-channel ECG device. This device can measure up to 14 days. The mean wear time was 7.6 ± 3.6 days. Compared with the first 48 h of monitoring, the overall diagnostic yield was greater compared to the one when data from the entire wear duration were included (62.2% vs. 43.9%).

As the characteristics of the Savvy sensor are equal or similar to the compared certified systems (see Table 6.1), the quality of the measured ECG by the Savvy sensor is expected to be equivalent. Because the Savvy sensor is rechargeable, the user can prolong the monitoring period by placing the sensor on different location on the body or use the sensor only when symptoms occur, which is not the case with one-time applicable devices (ZIO® XT patch, SEEQ™ sensor). On the other hand, the Savvy sensor can function only in tandem with a nearby smartphone/tablet, which may result in loss of ECG data if the smartphone/tablet is not close enough or is not functioning. Nevertheless, the opportunity to display real-time ECG data with the Savvy ECG system in many situations out-weights the "black box" concept of the ZIO® XT patch and the SEEQ™ sensor.

Safety
The main problem with prolonged ECG measurement is the sensitivity of the skin (skin irritation) to the compounds of the self-adhesive ECG electrodes. As was men-

Table 6.2 Skin problems from ECG patch devices

Question	Investigated users (%)
Wearing the monitoring system hurts	5
Wearing the monitoring system burns or stings	5
Wearing the monitoring system itches	45
Water bothers the monitoring system	17
My skin is irritated from wearing the monitoring system	43
My skin is sensitive from wearing the monitoring system	36
My skin bleeds from wearing the monitoring system	5

tioned previously, in a study with ZioPatch ECG monitoring [21] with 26751 patients, the mean wear time was 7.6 ± 3.6 days, although the ECG patch could measure up to 14 days. In the paper, there is no explanation of why the mean wear time was shorter than 14 days.

The results published in another study made by Ackermans et al. [22] can answer to the question above. They measured ECG up to 30 days with a 3-electrode skin patch with a detachable monitor device on 42 patients. The occurrence of skin problems as reported by patients for the investigated patch device is replicated from the study in Table 6.2.

As the user of the Savvy sensor can reposition the sensor to another location on the body, the serious problems with skin irritation can be diminished.

References

1. Ekeland, A., Bowes, A., Flottorp, S.: Effectiveness of telemedicine: a systematic review of reviews. Int. J. Med. Inform **79**, 736–771 (2010)
2. Rashkovska, A., Tomašić, I., Trobec, R.: A telemedicine application: ECG data from wireless body sensors on a smartphone. In: Proceedings of MEET & GVS on the 34th International Convention MIPRO 2011, vol. 1, pp. 293–296 (2011)
3. Sama, P.R., Eapen, Z.J., Weinfurt, K.P., Shah, B.R., Schulman, K.A.: An evaluation of mobile health application tools. JMIR mHealth uHealth **2**(2), e19 (2014)
4. Bort-Roig, J., Gilson, N.D., Puig-Ribera, A., Contreras, R.S., Trost, S.G.: Measuring and influencing physical activity with smartphone technology: a systematic review. Sports Med. **44**(5), 671–686 (2014)
5. EU, eHealth Ministerial Declaration, 22 may 2003. In: E-Health: Current Situation and Examples of Implemented and Beneficial E-Health Applications, IOS Press, Brussels, pp. 35–38 (2004)
6. Dzenowagis, J., Kernen, G.: Connecting for Health: Global Vision, Local Insight. Report for the World Summit on the Information Society, Geneva, Techical report, World Health Organization (2005)
7. WHO, eHealth Tools and Services: Needs of the Member States. Report of the Global Observatory for eHealth (2006)
8. Villani, A., Malfatto, G., Rosa, F.D., Rella, V., Comotti, T., Branzi, G., Compare, A., Bellardita, L., Molinari, E., Parati, G.: Clinical and psycological telemonitoring and telecare of high risk patients with chronic heart failure through wireless technologies: the icaros project. J. Clin. Exp. Cardiolog. **4**(8), 260 (2013)
9. Trobec, R., Avbelj, V., Meglič, B., Švigelj, V.: Analysis of baroreflex sensitivity. In: Proceedings of IASTED Conference on Biomedical Engineering, pp. 276–281 (2006)
10. Mohorčič, M., Depolli, M.: Heart rate analysis with NevroEkg. In: Proceedings of MEET & GVS on the 39th International Convention MIPRO, pp. 487–492 (2016)
11. Trobec, R., Avbelj, V., Rashkovska, A.: Multi-functionality of wireless body sensors. IPSI BgD Trans. Internet Res. **10**, 23–27 (2014)
12. Trobec, R., Depolli, M., Avbelj, V.: Wireless network of bipolar body electrodes. In: Seventh International Conference on Wireless On-demand Network Systems and Services (WONS), pp 145–150 (2010)
13. Bregar, K., Avbelj, V.: Multi-functional wireless body sensor—analysis of autonomy. In: Proceedings of MEET & GVS on the 36th International Convention MIPRO, pp. 346–349 (2013)
14. Trobec, R., Tomašić, I.: Synthesis of the 12-lead electrocardiogram from differential leads. IEEE Trans. Inf. Technol. Biomed. **15**(4), 615–621 (2011)

15. Tomašić, I., Frljak, S., Trobec, R.: Estimating the universal positions of wireless body electrodes for measuring cardiac electrical activity. IEEE Trans. Inf. Technol. Biomed. **60**(12), 3368–3374 (2013)
16. Trobec, R., Rashkovska, A., Avbelj, V.: Two proximal skin electrodes-a respiration rate body sensor. Sensors (Basel) **12**(10), 13813–13828 (2012)
17. Depolli, M., Avbelj, V., Trobec, R., Kališnik, J.M., Korošec, T., Susič, A.P., Stanič, U., Semeja, A.: PCARD platform for mHealth monitoring. Informatica **40**, 117–123 (2016)
18. Fung, E., Järvelin, M.-R., Doshi, R.N., Shinbane, J.S., Carlson, S.K., Grazette, L.P., Chang, P.M., Sangha, R.S., Huikuri, H.V., Peters, N.S.: Electrocardiographic patch devices and contemporary wireless cardiac monitoring. Front Physiol. **6**, 149 (2015)
19. Slak, J., Kosec, G.: Detection of heart rate variability from a wearable differential ECG device. In: Proceedings of Electronics and Microelectronics (MIPRO) 2016 39th International Convention Information and Communication Technology, pp. 430–435 (2016)
20. Barrett, P.M., Komatireddy, R., Haaser, S., Topol, S., Sheard, J., Encinas, J., Fought, A.J., Topol, E.J.: Comparison of 24-hour Holter monitoring with 14-day novel adhesive patch electrocardiographic monitoring. Am. J. Med. **127**(1), 95.e11–95.e17 (2014)
21. Turakhia, M.P., Hoang, D.D., Zimetbaum, P., Miller, J.D., Froelicher, V.F., Kumar, U.N., Xu, X., Yang, F., Heidenreich, P.A.: Diagnostic utility of a novel leadless arrhythmia monitoring device. Am. J. Cardiol. **112**, 520–524 (2013)
22. Ackermans, P.A., Solosko, T.A., Spencer, E.C., Gehman, S.E., Nammi, K., Engel, J., Russell, J.K.: A user-friendly integrated monitor-adhesive patch for long-term ambulatory electrocardiogram monitoring. J. Electrocardiol. **45**(2), 148–153 (2012)

Chapter 7
Final Remarks and Conclusions

Abstract The content of our book, devoted to body sensors and their implications to electrocardiography, is recapitulated with this chapter. The identified challenges in long-term ECG data analytics are discussed. Based on the presented material, the near future of mHealth perspectives is foreseen regarding the technology, the usability, and the potential of increased users' awareness for their own health.

7.1 Book Recapitulation

Improved medical care and increase in life conditions result in growth of the elderly population and a constant increase of healthcare costs. A breakthrough of ICT in health care could contribute to reduction in health-care costs in the near future, expecting the new generations of potential patients and medical personnel to accept new technologies on a day-to-day basis. The concept and technology of mHealth monitoring create basic changes in health services, focusing on the patient with personalized services and thus moving from curative to prevention. The mHealth can be regarded as a new way of supporting clinical health care at a distance, which is possible because of the readily available mobile infrastructures, small electronic devices and public communication options, like the Internet. The medical personnel can use communication on distance either for consulting and cooperation with their colleagues or for advising and guiding their patients at home.

The main motivations and goals of this book are presented in Chap. 1. The book has been motivated by challenges that arise from long-term ECG measurements required for reliable monitoring of the hearth rhythm during normal daily activities. In Chap. 2, we have presented how an unobtrusive medical-graded body sensor can be developed and implemented, using fundamental knowledge from multichannel ECG methodology. An adequate theoretical background for the differential lead used in the body ECG sensor is presented in Chap. 5. A distributed and complex computer software, presented in Chap. 3, is needed on different system levels, either as a firmware that enables a correct ECG data acquisition, or as a mobile application for the communication between the sensor and the mobile personal device, or as a personal computer program for visualization and analysis of the acquired ECG data.

© The Author(s) 2018   115
R. Trobec et al., *Body Sensors and Electrocardiography*, SpringerBriefs
in Applied Sciences and Technology, DOI 10.1007/978-3-319-59340-1_7

The described mHealth technology was first tested in laboratories to prove its applicability for medical use. We are grateful to many users of different profiles, patients and healthy volunteers, who have been engaged into several pilot measurements, some of them described in Chap. 4. Numerous comments and remarks have been obtained from the users and medical professionals, regarding affection to wearable devices and ECG measurements, social aspects, usability, medical value and others. The results and experiences regarding the technical aspects of research and development and those obtained from practical measurements confirm that body ECG sensors are a feasible solution for reliable and accurate long-term heart rhythm monitoring, which is crucial for the detection of various arrhythmias.

Already available sensors and associated mHealth services are presented in Chap. 6. Different approaches have been developed, from those to be used for 14 days and then returned to the clinic via mail, to those that offer online wireless transmission of data. Chest belt systems with wireless transmission are used in sports and for medical monitoring, where in the latter case at least bipolar-lead ECG signal with reasonable sampling accuracy is provided. These approaches are a step towards a future standard solution for long-term ECG monitoring, which is currently still not widely accepted. Although a single-channel bipolar ECG, e.g. a wearable ECG body sensor, carries less information than the standard 12-lead ECG, the latest findings indicate that, besides heart rhythm, some phenomena of the heart activity may be identified easier on a bipolar lead with a small distance between the electrodes. Therefore, it is even more important to bring such devices as close to the patients as possible.

The analysis of users' preferences, together with the exploitation of ICT and mobile infrastructures, can generate procedures and recommendations for improving the mHealth diagnostics evidence. They are briefly discussed in this chapter. The opportunities for larger clinical studies of chronic diseases could be significantly increased by aggregating the large amount of data obtained from the proposed monitoring. Remote medical care has a clear future as one of the regular medical care options, with mHealth being its leading economic and flexible technology.

7.2   Challenges in Long-Term ECG Analytics

The Holter monitor has been the standard for long-term ECG monitoring for more than 50 years. It is time to move forward, though, to follow the technological advances, and place wireless ECG monitoring devices in the healthcare system. One of the issues that are holding back the breakthrough of long-term sensor-based monitoring is the unavailability of methods for analysis of the acquired data. The methods for analysis are difficult to come by because they have to tackle the following crucial challenges:

- The state-of-the-art ECG analysis methods are tailored for the input from multichannel ECG equipment. In this type of equipment, more wired electrodes are used for signal acquisition. Usually, one to five leads are utilized for Holter ECG analysis, since multiple leads provide multiple viewpoints on the heart and provide redundancy that can be used in the analysis. The wireless body sensor, in contrast, acquires signal from a single differential lead that provides just a single viewpoint on the heart. However, more sensors can be used concurrently for a more detailed analysis.

- The lightweight design of Holter ECG, and in particular of wireless sensors, allows the patients to wear it comfortably for a long time and during their ordinary everyday activities. Since measurements are made on physically active subjects, the ECGs are more disturbed by baseline wandering and by missing data. The latter can occur on wireless sensors because the data is transmitted over a low-power radio connection with limited reliability. On the other hand, sensor ECG signals are less sensitive to electromagnetic interferences, if compared with Holter ECG signals, because sensor electrodes are placed close together.

- The wireless ECG body sensor is not always placed on the subject by a trained professional and can be miss-oriented. Furthermore, some skin irritation is an almost inevitable consequence of wearing the sensor for a long time because of the adhesive electrodes. Therefore, the analysis should be made possible for several different placements of sensors. Moreover, the users should have the option to interrupt long-term measurements for personal reasons, e.g. temporal reluctance to the measurement, showering, etc. These circumstances require that the analysis methods are robust to a wide range of ECG orientations and to the presence of noise in the recorded ECG.

- Finally, such devices are designed to be very energy efficient. Therefore, the measurements are sampled with a lower frequency, which helps conserve energy and prolong device autonomy. On the other hand, the long monitoring periods and the necessity for monitoring a large number of users concurrently, and in the real time, significantly increase the amount of data and the complexity of data analysis. Innovative approaches are needed for optimal preservation of data accuracy, management and analysis.

All of the above issues pose serious challenges for the adoption of currently existing analysis methods on the differential single-channel ECG measurements. New approaches are needed in the ECG data analytics, which will enable personalized analysis using knowledge extraction, deep learning, etc. The data analytics software for an mHealth system is laden with design challenges at every step. For the mHealth system to succeed, these challenges have to be met properly within the initial design. The challenge of ever-shifting user needs is also to be anticipated in case the mHealth system is accepted and welcomed by the general public. The impact of such mHealth system could also be broader than anticipated on a large number of connected medical areas. A successful mHealth system, however, seems to be within reach, as the technological challenges have been successfully met, while the software and social challenges certainly seem surmountable.

7.3 mHealth Perspectives

It is commonly considered that mHealth could decrease the costs of health care, offer higher equality in access to the health service and enable a personalized treatment based on long-term personal records, with the final goal of improving the quality of medical treatment. The use of mHealth technologies for data transfer can reduce the number of hospitalizations and thus reduce the burden on the entire healthcare system. An even wider impact can be considered, which includes lower energy consumption for the operation of the healthcare infrastructure and transport, lower operating costs, and reduction of negative environmental impact.

The mHealth technology has immensely improved over the last couple of years, primarily because of the great effort and amount of resources spent in development, and also because of the ever-developing and widely available mobile infrastructure worldwide. However, the benefit for the patients and healthy subjects is still small. Numerous solutions have been proposed for mHealth systems, both for the server side and for the sensors on the client side. However, a fully featured mHealth solution has not been yet accepted by a wide range of users. There are several reasons: technical, social and economic, why mHealth solutions are remaining a goal for the future instead of being an everyday reality. The diversity of users' needs, proprietary acquisition and communication protocols, obtrusive sensors, complicated usage, non-reliable measurements during physical activities, and reluctance to novelties are some of them. The main focus is currently on the use of sensor systems and protocols, which are mostly tailored for applications that improve well-being. New sensor systems for medical applications have a much higher potential for the optimization of healthcare systems and for reducing the inequalities in health service availability. Finally, in the actual implementation of a national mHealth system, a transparent and competitive inclusion of local innovative industry is required. Besides new bioengineering and medical experts, also specialized caregivers, especially for older users, should be educated.

Increasing the reliability and user friendliness of mHealth systems is the key prerequisite for further developments. The developments are stimulated by increase of the number of remotely monitored users on the account of a more cost-effective health care. For further developments and implementations, efforts should be focused on original and innovative paths for bringing the existing technologies closer to the users, and on including the users' immediate healthcare environment, e.g. their family, caregivers, friends and volunteers. Wider dissemination of mHealth services will enable self-management of diseases, increase of healthcare efficiency and minimization of the users' expenditure. The obtained knowledge from the medical-grade long-term ECG monitoring will contribute to the development of new diagnostic foundations for heart rhythm disturbances and possibly also for myocardial ischemia.

Emerging databases of measurements in Cloud data storage offer a unique opportunity for scientific exploration and advances in medical knowledge on the national level, e.g. epidemic studies. ECG measurements that are several days long and are enriched with subject's activity data will be available in large quantity, and will provide the input for a new research frontier. Although processing this data will be difficult, the state-of-the-art Bigdata techniques are rapidly approaching the required level of maturity for being able to tackle the challenge. The research of the documented data and information will feed back the new knowledge into updates and new designs of mHealth systems that will benefit the mHealth users almost immediately. If we extrapolate the current trend, we can foresee that mHealth services will become one of the fastest growing industries for collective benefits.

Index

© The Author(s) 2018
R. Trobec et al., *Body Sensors and Electrocardiography*, SpringerBriefs
in Applied Sciences and Technology, DOI 10.1007/978-3-319-59340-1

Printed in the United States
By Bookmasters